Mommy, My Head Hurts

are really sick? Do you think people die sometimes from headaches like yours?

- What does (mom, dad, sister, brother, etc.) think of your headaches?
- When you have a headache, do you think about it a lot? Do you wonder if it will get worse? Or do you just wait for it to get better on its own?

If your child admits to worrying about his headaches, to having sadness or other feelings because of them, be sympathetic. Let your child know that everybody feels the way he does some of the time, and encourage him to continue talking to you about his thoughts.

It may take several times asking these questions before you get a response, and you may have to ask them several different ways, but be both patient and persistent. However, some of these questions may not be appropriate for your particular child. You should tailor the questions to your child, his personality, and your particular situation.

Children aged seven to eleven do understand that pains tend to have a specific cause, and along with this increased understanding comes a realization that headache pain could also represent serious illness. They may still echo earlier ways of thinking and believe that the headaches are there because they have done something wrong. Moreover, children of this age group can become frightened as they realize that the headache could potentially represent serious illness or even death. This becomes worse if they see their parents frightened as well. Because of their feelings of fear, they may exaggerate their symptoms to get more attention from their parents.

It is especially important for parents to realize this and tailor their response to the headache appropriately. Parents need to be able to deal with their child's pain and anxiety in a low-key, matter-of-fact way. Their words and body language need to convey support and acknowledgement of their child's pain, but must not play into or amplify their child's fears. For this to happen, parents do need to feel comfortable that their child's headaches are not due to a serious underlying problem. Addressing this concern specifically with your child's doctor will help you to feel secure about this.

Once parents feel at ease, they must communicate this specifically to their child, especially if the child's doctor has not. Look your child in the eye and say, "You are healthy, but you are having headaches. You don't feel good when you have headaches, but it doesn't mean that anything is terribly wrong with you. You are going to be OK." Your child will then know that you are there for him, that you are confident that he will soon feel better, and that you are not worried about him. Your child will view himself as someone healthy with a temporary pain rather than viewing himself as a sickly person who is not expected to recover. You are also sending a clear message to him that he cannot "use" your worry to get *extra* attention for his headaches.

In a related true-life example, one child's headaches improved remarkably, simply by bringing up these issues. Michael was ten years old, and had always been what his mother termed a "sensitive" child. He always seemed to think about everything more than his happy-go-lucky younger sister. In fourth grade now, he was a great student, and outside of school he seemed very happy with playing on the computer and karate classes. He came from an intact family and there were no apparent problems in his home life. In the spring, he developed headaches that got worse and worse, keeping him out of school about ten days a month and causing him to miss a lot of the activities that had previously given him so much pleasure. Although he'd been having headaches off and on over the past two years, his parents became quite alarmed at the changes they were seeing and felt convinced that their child must have a brain tumor. Michael's maternal grandfather had in fact died of a brain tumor about five

Mommy, My Head Hurts

A Doctor's Guide to Your Child's Headaches

SARAH CHEYETTE, M.D.

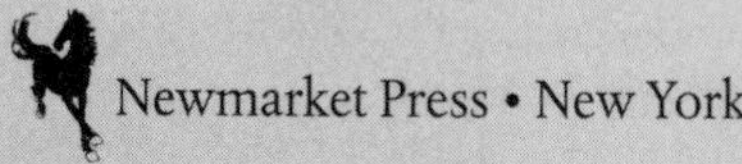
Newmarket Press • New York

FIRST EDITION

Library of Congress Cataloging-in-Publication Data

Cheyette, Sarah

Mommy, my head hurts : a doctor's guide to your child's headaches / by Sarah Cheyette.—1st ed.

p. cm.

1. Headache in children. I. Title.

RJ496.H3 C477 2001 2001026680

618.92'8491—dc21 CIP

ISBN 1-55704-471-6

QUANTITY PURCHASES

Companies, professional groups, clubs, and other organizations may qualify for special terms when ordering quantities of this title. For information, write Special Sales, Newmarket Press, 18 East 48th Street, New York, NY 10017, call (212) 832-3575, fax (212) 832-3629, or e-mail mailbox@newmarketpress.com.

www.newmarketpress.com

Manufactured in the United States of America

10 9 8 7 6 5 4 3 2 1

This book contains the opinions and ideas of its author. It is designed to provide accurate and authoritative information in regard to the subject matter covered. It is published with the understanding that the author and publisher are not engaged in rendering medical, health, or any other kind of personal professional services in the book. The reader should consult his or her medical, health, or other competent professional before adopting any of the suggestions in this book or drawing inferences from it.

The author and publisher specifically disclaim all responsibility for any liability, loss, or risk, personal or otherwise, that is incurred as a consequence, directly or indirectly, of the use and application of any of the contents of this book.

To my husband, Ben, and my children Madeleine and Natalie, for their love, support, inspiration, and delight.

Special thanks to my parents, professors, and patients, for their guidance, and to Dr. Jong Rho for very helpful comments on the manuscript.

Contents

Foreword

In *Mommy, My Head Hurts: A Doctor's Guide to Your Child's Headaches,* Dr. Cheyette has given parents a wonderfully clear, complete, current text on headaches and their treatment. This information will give all parents the chance to go through the same routine that their child's doctor uses in coming to a diagnosis and course of therapy for their child. The book gives clear insight on when they will need to consult with their child's physician and will allow them to ask more insightful questions of their doctor. This will enable a quicker diagnosis and treatment to occur and should help bring more rapid relief to the child. I sincerely recommend this book by Dr. Cheyette to all parents of children with headaches (as Dr. Cheyette points out—almost all parents) and to their physicians as well.

Dr. Donald E. Cook,
President, American Academy of Pediatarics

Introduction

You are reading this book for a simple reason: your child has been in pain, and you want to help him or her.

I am writing this book for several reasons. First and foremost, I believe that the problem of headaches in children is enormous, but has been underappreciated for a variety of reasons. I would like to give the children (and their affected families) more of a voice. Second, as a parent of two young children, I am sympathetic to the concerns and anxieties of parents caring for their children.

Headache causes about four and a half lost school days per child every year, and 40 percent of all children have had at least one headache by age seven, according to a 1994 Centers for Disease Control (CDC) report. However, there is very little information available on the specific needs of children who suffer headaches.

I specialized in neurology, first as a resident and then in private practice, and I have seen hundreds of children with headaches, some quite severe and some less so. I have been impressed by the complexity of dealing with a child who has headaches, as there are so many factors involved. There are the medical causes of and treatments for the headache, but in addition a number of psychological and social factors are also involved. The impact of the psychological and social factors can be enormous, sometimes outweighing the medical aspects in determining the impact of the headaches on the child's life.

The fact that the headaches are occurring in children makes them even more challenging to treat than the headaches that adults suffer. For example, children, with their limited verbal abilities and experience, may have difficulty communicating what they are feeling during a headache. They may appear very ill, with no outward sign of what is happening to them. Their parents need guidance in helping them through their headaches. Sadly, to date there has been very little published regarding headaches in children. Addressing this lack of information was really the impetus to write this book. The aim of this book is to give parents the knowledge they need to best manage their child's headaches.

Much of the information available to parents about children's headaches comes from books that focus on adult headaches and that have only a few pages on children. This, however, is inadequate. Children deserve a book that takes into account their particular issues—issues that are less relevant for adults. For example, how do children of different ages think about pain? How do the headaches affect their interactions with their parents and siblings? What treatments are particularly effective in children?

Headaches can represent a complicated problem for so many children and their families. In my office practice, I do attempt to cover all aspects that need to be discussed, but I am often limited by time constraints. This book is a way for me to discuss the complexity of my patients' problems in the manner that I feel they deserve.

Headaches are a subject that can engender fear in both parents and medical care practitioners alike. There is something mysterious about a force that causes so much pain, yet leaves no outward marks. Headaches conjure up fears of brain tumors and other serious medical illnesses, especially in an otherwise healthy young child. Yet for the vast majority of child headache sufferers, the headaches are treatable and not associated with death or disability. I hope that this book alleviates some of the fear for both parents and their children.

It is my goal here to give you, the reader, a better understanding of your child's headaches. I hope the knowledge you gain will be a comfort to you. Knowledge is also power, and this book is intended to make you feel more in control of a difficult situation. Use it, with the medical resources available to you, to help your child.

Mommy,
My Head Hurts

CHAPTER 1

I Have an Owie!
The Concept of Pain in a Child

"Owie. Owie. Owie!" —*Josh, three years old*

"It just hurts!" —*Alexa, eight years old*

"It feels like somebody is taking my head and squeezing it between two bricks!" —*Alyssa, thirteen years old*

Headaches are, of course, a type of pain. Therefore, to really understand headaches in children, we must first think about how children understand and talk about pain.

As adults, we perceive pain very differently than children do. For one thing, we tend to think of pain as very objective, as something that has a direct relationship to the amount of damage done to the body. A papercut, for example, only hurts a little bit, while cutting yourself with a steak knife hurts more, and so on. We assume that each situation causes a measurable amount of pain that most people would agree on.

Pain in a child seems to be less related to the actual amount of damage. For a child, many factors enter into the amount he suffers from pain. Age plays a major role. Gender may also be involved. Prior experiences with pain that he has had will influence him. What she is doing at the time of the headache is a factor. How his parents react to and deal with the pain is also important. All of these issues seem to be more important in how a child interprets and responds to pain as compared to an adult.

Headache pain may be even more difficult for a child to process than other types of pain. After all, if you suffer a hurt by cutting yourself, you will see something—blood. If your finger is painful because of an infection, you will see something—swelling and redness—and you can touch it. Everyone who has been in these situations will be able to look at the child and understand: *oh yeah, that hurts a lot.* In these cases, something is obviously wrong, something that a child can point to and that adults can see. But what about headaches, which cannot be seen or touched by a child and the adults around him?

This chapter will help you to understand different factors involved in your child's pain. This greater awareness will give you a greater ability to help your child.

PAIN—DEFINED

When asked, "what is pain?" children of different ages will give you different definitions, and these definitions are different from those an adult will give. Pain is not, however, an easy word for anybody to define.

Even adults who study the subject have difficulty verbally defining pain better than my eight-year-old patient Andrew, who said "Pain is something that hurts." Compare this to the "official" definition. A group called The International Association for the Study of Pain defined pain as an unpleasant sensory and emotional experience associated with actual or potential tissue damage—loosely translated, what you feel when you get hurt. The most important part of their definition is that it recognizes that pain has both sensory and emotional components to it, both of which are important.

However, these definitions emphasize "getting hurt." It is harder to apply this concept to headaches than it is to a visible wound of some sort (such as major surgery or pain felt after an automobile accident, for example).

Choosing Your Words About Pain Carefully

It is hard for anybody to really understand and define the word "pain" and the meaning behind it. Adults have a fuller, more robust understanding of pain than children do. So as an adult dealing with a child who is in pain, try to use a child's words and concepts rather than your own. For example, in questioning a young child who needs concrete words about his pain, "point to where it hurts your head," is much more likely to lead to an answer than "tell me about your pain."

Similarly, be careful about the words you use to talk to your child about the pain. Don't say, "Nothing's wrong." Something is wrong, or your child would not be acting differently, and he may then increase the behaviors he displays with his pain (crying, lack of activity, etc.) in an attempt to convince you. If you don't feel your child is actually feeling as much pain as he is telling you about, don't negate his feelings by denying them. Instead, focus on the process of getting better: "You'll feel better soon."

Children's perception of what hurts changes as they get older. During the developmental process, they gain new and more complex ways of thinking and more experience with the world around them. Therefore, as they grow, how they react to painful experiences changes.

Younger children, two to six years old, tend to focus on the simple sensory aspect of the pain. Children this age use words like "owie" or "boo-boo" to describe all their hurts. Tiny scrapes are, to them, as significant as major wounds. They focus on the more concrete aspects, such as what can be seen on their skin after a scrape, rather than the more abstract "pain."

As children get older they develop more experience with pain. They have lived through scraped knees, scabs big and small, cuts, stitches, broken bones, and falling off bikes. They are able to compare current pains to previous ones, and their previous pains become the basis for defining how much the current ones hurt. They can recognize that the pain of a broken arm was worse than the time they stepped on glass, and that large amounts of damage are more painful than small ones. They have greater language abilities and are better able to describe the different aspects of their pain.

Especially during the teenage years, but even before, children are more likely to include emotional factors in their definition of pain as well as physical aspects. For teenagers, the emotional component is often at least as important as the physical experience of pain. They understand that pain can make you sad and anxious, and that these feelings are often as uncomfortable as the physical pain itself.

As our children grow, we must take into account their changing viewpoints. The next few sections will discuss pain from infancy to adolescence, focusing on the developmental issues.

DO INFANTS GET HEADACHES?

We don't know how an infant relates to pain. Surprisingly, only recently has there been recognition that infants could feel pain at all. It was believed that their nervous systems were not mature enough to process pain, and that many of the behavioral responses to pain (grimacing and crying, for example) were a result of fear rather than pain. As a mother, I was especially shocked to find that the subject of pain in children did not begin to be addressed until the 1970s, and even for ten years after that there was not much interest. People thought that babies neither perceived pain nor remembered it, and so the possibility of pain in babies was generally ignored. There were also concerns about the dangers of giving anesthetics to infants. Babies who underwent operations—the same types of operations given to adults who received loads of potent pain medications—did so without the benefit of medications to relieve pain, even undergoing the operations without anesthesia. Editorials in the popular press by a mother whose premature baby underwent an hour-and-a-half operation without anesthesia in 1986 were fundamental in bringing the issue to public attention.

The people who were working with these children were not monsters, but their thinking was based on assumptions that babies can't perceive or remember pain, assumptions we now recognize as wrong. However this recognition was slow in coming. Even during my training in the early 1990s, when my fellow residents and I were learning to perform circumcisions on newborn baby boys, we asked about pain medications for them. "Don't worry," we were told, "it's quick and they won't remember it anyway." Even when pain medications were given, children were often under-dosed. Many physicians were—and still are—uncomfortable with giving such potent medicines to babies because of fear of overdosing them.

Medical concepts eventually changed, however, and it is now clear that even well before they are born, infant nervous systems are developed enough to be physically capable of transmitting pain messages. Studies have also convinced people that babies remember pain, as well; babies as young as six months will learn to avoid something that has previously caused them pain. So at least we are now recognizing that babies do experience pain, learn from it, and remember it. But what of the emotional component to pain, the subjective feelings associated with it? Like many aspects of infancy, what a baby is actually feeling and thinking about is often a mystery.

So babies experience pain. Do they experience headaches? It is unclear at what age headaches begin. In the books and articles written about babies' experience of pain, headaches are generally not mentioned. It is clear that babies are uncomfortable when they have meningitis (an infection around the brain, which is very painful in older children and adults), so they are probably capable of experiencing pain from other causes of headaches as well. However, we really don't know when headaches start. One report claimed that infants as young as four months could suffer from migraines. The study looked retrospectively at children when they were older, and had their parents think back to episodes that could have been headaches in infancy. For example, a child who at the age of two had clear episodes of headache and vomiting had episodes of otherwise unexplained vomiting as young as four months. At two, these vomiting episodes were thought to be associated with a headache disorder. However, at the time the child was four months, nobody could have known that the episodes represented headaches.

We do know now that by age two some children experience headaches. Most two-year-old children are quite capable of saying, "it hurts," or "head hurts." However, this does not mean that they understand pain in the same way as an adult might perceive it, although they use similar words.

PRESCHOOLERS AND THEIR "OWIES" (AGES TWO THROUGH SIX)

Again, there is shockingly little information regarding preschoolers and their responses to pain, despite the fact that preschoolers incontrovertibly feel pain and are developing concepts about it. Pain is a real issue in children of this age, and how they develop their concepts of pain could potentially influence how they deal with pain for the rest of their lives. Those of us who are parents and those of us who work with children this age have made a number of observations that guide us in understanding pain as they experience it. We can use these observations to help guide our management of the pain.

At the ages of two and three, most preschoolers become quite interested in their bodies. They are learning new skills such as jumping or how to do a somersault. They are climbing all over things, running very fast, and consequently suffering lots of scrapes, bruises, and bumps. It is typically these little episodes of pain, or small "owies," that prompt children to begin to think about, and therefore talk about, pain.

These small owies, though a little painful at the time, can carry great rewards. The rewards often overshadow the amount of pain involved. "Owies" carry with them associations of adults fussing over them, giving them hugs and kisses to take away their pain, and the opportunity to play with that fascinating substance, ice. Children this age can really learn to "turn on" the tears when they get hurt; it may start out as genuine, but can quickly become a habit used to gain attention. Here's a situation that should be familiar to all parents:

> Alison, two years old, sobs after she bumps her head getting out of the car. "It hurts, mommy," she says and continues to sob.
>
> Alison's mommy says, "Here's a kiss to make it all better." She kisses Alison's head. "Is it all better now?"
>
> A moment later, Alison says, "All better," and immediately turns to do something else.

The pain can be replayed whenever sympathy is needed. Trevor, pointing to a scab a week old, will still say, "It hurts me."

My daughter, age three, knows she will get ice if she gets an owie. Like most preschoolers, she is quite intrigued with ice: the temperature of it is different from most things she comes across, its shape changes, it is fun to eat. So for her, having an owie has the benefit of getting a bag of ice to play with. When she gets a bump, one of the first things she says is, "I have an owie, I need ice." Only it sounds like, "IhaveanowieIneedICE!" she is in such a hurry to get to the ice.

Children this age have the need to delineate certain items as their own ("That's my doll!" "That's my fork!"), and along with this comes the need to have what others have. The subject of owies is no exception. Children this age are quite fascinated by their skin, which is where the visible reminders of these little owies are most apparent. Their skin breaks, changes color, and is something they can point to and show everybody to indicate what they have been through. If one child in a group points out an owie on their skin, the other children in the group will point out their owies, real or imagined, with great gusto.

Here's a conversation recently overheard on a playground, as a group of two-and-a-half to three year olds were in the sandbox:

"I have an owie," said Alexandra.

"No, I have an owie," Lisa said.

"I have TWO owies," Alexandra said, as her voice began to rise.

"I have TWO owies," Lisa returned.

"I have an owie over there," another child, Hannah, said as she joined in, pointing to her clearly healthy arm.

"I have an owie over there, TOO." Alexandra was getting quite angry, and she walked over and gave Hannah an owie (a slap on her shoulder).

Children this age are learning that the owies can come as a consequence of actions, actions that they may or may not have initiated, but for which there is a cause-and-effect relationship. For example, a child could get hurt because he ran and fell, or because another child pulled his hair; either way, there is pain linked to a particular activity. Establishing cause and effect has some benefits; the child will potentially remember the pain associated with the running and slow down, thereby keeping the child safer. However, children this age do not have a well-defined understanding of consequences. They will look to anything in the immediate environment that they associate with pain as an explanation, not necessarily the cause of their accident. So, the child who fell while running might point to a nearby table on which he had previously bumped his head as the cause of his pain, rather than the fact that he was moving too quickly. Although they may not always get the cause of the pain correct, children this age do look hard for reasons.

A negative consequence of getting owies is the pain involved, but for most children the incidents of pain are short-lived and minor. Children who have repetitively suffered minor pain will not understand, in times of more severe pain, why Mommy can't kiss it away. They are used to episodes of pain being short and ending with something nice. Children who start to develop headaches, which often last longer and are more severe than their little owies, have not developed a concept of time. They do not understand that some pains take longer to go away than others, despite Mommy's kisses.

After all, when Mommy gives sympathy, preschoolers may invest her actions with a magical ability to take away pain. Children, especially those in the two-and-a-half to four-year range, are naturally imaginative and magical in their thinking. They have imaginary friends who are quite real to them. They can become a fireman or a ballerina in the blink of an eye. A cardboard box may become a racecar, only to be changed a moment later into an airplane. They have a strong tendency to form an association between dissimilar events that enter their perception, solely because they occur together, whereas older children and adults turn to logic as a way to associate things. Therefore, preschoolers associate Mommy's kisses, ice, or other forms of attention with the actual taking away of the pain, although older children know that logically these things do not affect the actual healing process.

Similarly, older children may logically reason that the pain of headaches can be attributed to internal factors: my head hurts because I have migraines, because my neck muscles are tight, etc.

Preschool children don't have a clue what goes on inside their bodies; they are much more focused on the outsides of them. So a preschooler is more likely to invent a magical rule—almost a superstitious reason—why they have a headache: for example, maybe they got the headache because they misbehaved. Some children extend this logic and think, Maybe I misbehaved, and so maybe I shouldn't tell anybody about my headache. Preschoolers are also likely to point to the tummy as the source of all pain, for reasons that nobody really understands.

Children are egocentric at the preschool age, meaning that their whole world revolves around themselves. This egocentrism certainly plays a role in their ability to communicate their pain to other people. Children of this age have trouble understanding that their thoughts are distinct from other people's and that other people cannot read their minds; they may assume that what they are thinking, other people are thinking, too. Therefore, they may not communicate their pain to others, thinking that others already know about it.

They are also developing a very strong sense of control, most evident in the area of potty training but also in the increasing need to "do it myself." When they are in pain, they lose control, which becomes quite scary for them. The negative feelings they experience about losing control may be, for them, as bad as the actual pain of the experience itself. Therefore, giving children of this age a sense of control over their pain is one of the most helpful things an adult can do for them.

Headache pain must be particularly hard on preschoolers given these developmental considerations. They leave no visible marks for the preschoolers to look at (and brag about later). Adults cannot see the cause of the pain, and the preschoolers may not understand why the adults don't automatically understand what they are experiencing. The headaches come without a defined cause, and no one—not even Mommy—can control them and make them vanish.

PAIN IN SEVEN TO ELEVEN YEAR OLDS

In this age group, children are capable of thinking about pain in a more logical and precise way than when they were younger. For example, they are more verbal and can describe it more clearly. They can localize the pain more accurately to different parts of their head, and for the first time can describe details about it, such as a feeling of tightness or pounding. This can be a great help to parents and the doctor. Below are two typical conversations I might have in my office about headaches, one with an eight year old, and one with a four year old. Compare the two:

Doctor to eight-year-old Erik: "Can you tell me a little about your headache? Can you point to where it hurts?"

Erik, pointing to his forehead: "It hurts here. And when it hurts, it feels like someone is pushing my head tight."

Doctor to four-year-old Matt: "Can you point to where your head hurts?"

Matt just looks at his mom.

Children in the older age group are more aware of some of the emotional feelings that can accompany episodes of pain, such as sadness or anxiety. As they begin to understand these accompanying feelings, they can begin to understand that sometimes dealing with the feelings is as important as dealing with the underlying pain. They are able to talk about the feelings, so it is important to ask about them.

Doctor to nine-year-old Samantha (who had been having headaches almost every day for a month): "Samantha, you have missed a lot of fun things because of your headaches. What do you think about that?"

Samantha: "Sometimes it makes me sad, and I want the headaches to go away."

Doctor: "What do you think your mom thinks about when you have a headache?"

Samantha: "I think she's worried about me, and wants to make me feel better."

Doctor: "Are there any good things about having headaches so much?"

Samantha: "Sometimes I don't have to put the dishes away."

Questions to ask your seven- to eleven-year-old child about his headaches

Conversations like these don't have to be limited to the doctor's office, and in fact are probably better done by the parents. At home, children will probably speak more freely than they do in the doctor's office. I get a lot of "I don't know" answers, which is the most frequent response a child will give when he really does know, but doesn't want to tell me. Here are some questions you can ask your child to try to understand how he feels about the headaches. These questions become more and more important to ask if headaches are getting worse or are occurring more frequently. The answers may not only surprise you, but may also give you important clues to managing the headaches.

- How do you feel when your headaches make you miss something fun?
- How do you feel when your headaches make you miss school?
- Sometimes people get headaches because they worry a lot about different things. Does that sound like you?
- Sometimes people can think of good parts about having headaches, like extra attention from mom, and not having to do some things like cleaning your room. Can you think of any good parts about your headaches?
- When you get a headache, do you think that it means you

years earlier. They made an appointment with their physician, and in the week before the appointment the headaches got particularly bad. Michael's activity level plummeted, and he spent a lot of time just lying on the couch.

It turned out that Michael had heard a story about a friend's father who had died of cancer, and one of his symptoms had been head pain. Michael was worried that his head pain meant that he also had cancer, or something else bad, and when his parents were clearly worried about him this validated his concerns. If his parents were worried about him, it must be true. Every time he had the slightest bit of headache it signaled to him that he must really be sick. In the week before the appointment with the doctor, his parents were quite anxious and so was Michael.

At their appointment the doctor was able to convince Michael and his parents that Michael was in fact OK. Just hearing that he was not suffering from anything serious was a tremendous relief to Michael, and his headaches largely cleared up without any medications. He still got them once in a while, but was able to go on about his usual business.

When you are letting your child know that he will be all right even if he has headaches, be sure that you also tell his siblings. Children of this age often have siblings who can have their own fears about their brother's or sister's headaches. It is important that they get the same message: everything is going to be just fine, and the headaches are just going to be something that we will deal with together.

Overall, in this age group children do not like it when their headaches interfere with their normal activities. They want to continue with their usual routine, and only rarely will consciously use their headache to get out of chores or schoolwork. Parents often ask if they should make their child lie down when he has a headache, or let him do his activity. My advice is that as much as possible, normal routines should not be interrupted. If your child is in so much pain that the normal routine is clearly impossible, he should be treated with understanding but with firm guidelines. For example, if your child has a headache that prevents him from cleaning his room, he needs to lie down in a quiet room *without* television or other entertainment; he should not be allowed to play video games instead. This will prevent the headaches from being tied in subconsciously or consciously to pleasurable experiences. In and of itself, without medications, this approach may help to significantly decrease the frequency of your child's headaches.

TWELVE AND OLDER: HEADACHES IN THE TEENAGE YEARS

Teenagers are, of course, famous for *causing* headaches in their parents. In turn, most physicians will agree that taking care of teenagers who have headaches involves special challenges as well. What is going on with your teenager at this time of his life?

Children at this stage become proficient at abstract thinking. They are able to relate to pain in a more conceptual way, rather than focusing on the concrete way it feels. That is, they are getting away from the focus on "it hurts," and becoming able to understand pain in a more complex way. The focus on pain can shift almost entirely from the physical aspects to the emotional aspects; teenagers tend to describe pain in terms of their emotional response to it: "It's awful, it's unbearable, I don't like it." Pain is recognized as having psychological consequences such as anxiety, and teenagers are readily able to understand that anxiety and stress can contribute to headaches.

By this stage, teenagers have more experience with pain. Simply because they have lived through more years than younger children, there is more of a chance that they have suffered severe pains, such as from broken bones. They can compare the current pain of their headaches to previous painful experiences: which hurts more and which hurts less, for example. They can compare headache pain to the pain of major injuries, as well as compare one headache to another one they had suffered in the past. The ability to compare pains over time can play a role in terms of the amount of anxiety a pain experience can generate. A teenager (or adult) is less likely to be concerned about her headache if she recognizes it as something that has happened many times in the past, as something she got through all of those times with no permanent problems. In contrast, a headache pain that is felt to be above and beyond all that she has previously experienced is (understandably) more likely to cause stress.

Stress can play an enormous role in how and why teenagers have headaches. Teenagers are already suffering through a lot of "natural" stresses because of the developmental conflicts that arise during those years. Specifically, two major issues play a role in how teenagers deal with the pain of headaches. First, teenagers are struggling between a strong drive toward independence versus a need for security and support. With health issues such as headaches, this conflict plays into a clash between wanting the nurturing and loving that parents had previously supplied during times of illness and the desire to handle things on their own. Part of them wants Mommy to kiss it, the other part wants Mom to just go away.

A second conflict involves how teenagers view their bodies in general. Despite a need to "develop into my own person" and become an individual, most teens at this stage want nothing more than to just be like everybody else. They want to dress like everyone else, and they want to look like every one else. Bodies become a major focus for teens: not just looking at other people's bodies, but carefully scrutinizing one's own. They want their bodies to be just the same, but headaches (and other illnesses) can become a major disruption to their plans. Any changes in or talk about their bodies can cause a great deal of embarrassment. In a doctor's office, teens are the most likely group to clam up (they may, on their talkative days, squeeze out an "I don't know" on occasion) despite the fact that they probably spend a great deal of time thinking about their headaches in private. They become more focused on their headaches as compared to their responses in earlier years, just as they are more focused on their bodies in general.

Teens are under general physical stress as well. This is a time when their bodies are growing at tremendous rates, and hormones are exploding in ways not previously experienced. These physical changes, hormones foremost, are in and of themselves likely to contribute to headaches. For some females, migraines clearly are influenced by their monthly cycles. Statistically, girls are more likely to develop migraines at the onset of puberty than at any other time in their lives (see Chapter 3). In contrast, boys (whose migraines are more likely to start prepubertally) may at this stage experience some improvement in their symptoms.

Depression is also recognized as commonly occurring in the teenage years, for reasons that are unclear. This is so serious that every year more than 4 percent of ninth graders in the United States make suicide attempts serious enough to require medical attention. Is this a natural physiologic consequence of pubertal changes of brain chemistry, or are other external stress factors making more of a contribution? Especially in this day and age, teenagers are more likely to have suffered through one or more parental divorces and may have also been exposed to adult-themed problems in school such as drugs, pregnancy, violence, and the like. In any case, depression and headaches can go hand in hand. Often, we don't know if the depression causes the headaches, or if the headaches contribute to depression. Both headaches and depression do involve some common neurotransmitters (chemicals which brain cells use to communicate with each other), most notably serotonin (see Chapter 2 for more details). How teenagers deal with their headaches can affect overall depression, and vice versa.

Here is an example of a teenager with, as he put it, "a major headache problem."

Brandon, fifteen years old, had suffered occasional headaches, but none that had particularly slowed him down until recently. Now in the spring of ninth grade, he had progressively been missing more and more school because of his headaches. He had gotten to the point where his headache never stopped; it was there all the time. His primary medical care provider had tried a number of different medications, but none provided more than mild and temporary relief, and everyone was getting discouraged. Brandon first had a computerized tomography (CT) scan, then a magnetic resonance imaging (MRI) scan, both of which were entirely normal.

After a couple of weeks of going to school about half-time, leaving early many days, Brandon began to spend most of his days at home. He would stay up until about midnight and sleep in until about 11 A.M. He did not exercise because he felt it worsened his headache. He watched a lot of television and spent time surfing the web as well. He saw his friends on occasion, but certainly not as much as he used to, and he "didn't really feel" like doing much with them anyway. His parents arranged to have homework assignments sent home from school, most of which Brandon did, but he could not really keep up with his classes. His school began to talk about holding him back a year. Brandon, already somewhat withdrawn, became more so after hearing the news. He really felt helpless to change the situation. His parents, too, were at their wits' end. They did not know what to do to improve things.

Everyone felt a little better after seeing the neurologist, because after examining Brandon and talking to him and his parents, the neurologist was able to reassure them that Brandon did not have a disease that was being missed. Although he could not give them any immediate solutions, the doctor and family came up with a plan to be implemented over the next month or two.

Brandon was started on a daily medication to try to lessen the daily headache, and he was given some other medications to try if the headache became particularly bad. He was given some relaxation exercises to do every day and a referral to a formal biobehavioral program. He was also asked to get himself "reconditioned" for school: getting back to the wake/sleep cycle that he would need to follow to get to morning classes and beginning a very modest exercise program.

After a couple of weeks, there was not much difference. Some additional medication adjustments were made, but mainly Brandon was asked to hang in there, and he was given some positive feedback for some changes that indicated he was heading in the right direction. He began biobehavioral training and felt it helped him. In the program, issues involving stress and depression were more fully explored. Brandon and his parents went through some counseling sessions, but Brandon was not thought to be clinically depressed.

Finally Brandon was able to go back to school, first part time and finally, full time. He had one relapse two years later, but generally headaches were better controlled, and he was taken off much of his medication over the next two to three years.

OTHER FACTORS THAT MAY BE INFLUENCING YOUR CHILD'S PAIN

The previous sections have discussed how your child's age may have an influence on how headaches affect his life. However, there are other factors that can play a role. Age is probably the most important factor in how your child responds to his headaches, but the following aspects can also be important.

Gender. Although there has been some controversy on this issue, most studies seem to indicate that the physical process of feeling pain probably is not much different whether the child suffering the pain is a girl or a boy. That is, girls and boys feel the same amount of pain if they suffer the same injury: a papercut is just as likely to give an "owie" in a girl or a boy. However, girls and boys may react differently to the pain. A girl may be more likely to talk about the pain, and may be more likely to react to pain by taking medicine for it. Differences in how boys and girls react to pain most likely reflect cultural influences.

For example, families may also give different responses to boys and girls who are in pain. Sally might be encouraged to rest and take ibuprofen if she has a stomachache, whereas her brother Jack might be told that it'll be over soon and he will be fine. Families' reactions translate into cues for their children about how to react to pain. In this example, Sally is essentially being told that the way to deal with her pain is to rest and take medication, whereas her brother Jack is being taught to work through it. Over time and with the various pain issues that come up, these cues get reinforced over and over, and they will shape the way Sally and Jack react to new painful experiences in the future.

Your Child's Personality. Children who have recurrent headaches tend to be over-achievers, expecting perfection of themselves. They therefore tend to set themselves up for stress and frustration when things don't go the way they want them to go. They may be more focused on their body, expecting perfection there and therefore interpreting any sign of pain as a major problem. You may be able to help your child's headaches by helping him understand and set more realistic goals for himself.

Family. One of the most important factors in how a child responds to pain comes from the family. From infancy, a child is surrounded by parents and other family members who react when the child gets hurt. Some parents will react to their toddler's bumps and bruises with a huge display of emotion:

"Did Johnny bump his head on the table? Oh, my poor little boy, let me kiss it, oh my baby." Others will take a more low-key tact: "Be more careful next time." Families generally are more protective and upset by injuries to their first-born children than the later-born children, and interestingly there is research to indicate that first-born children are more sensitive to pain. Families will also react differently to pain in younger children than pain in older ones. Younger children are more likely to receive supportive kisses and bandages for scrapes than are older children.

I think my child is "faking it." What should I do?

You never want to discount your child's pain, especially because you can't really tell exactly what he is experiencing. However, if you are pretty sure that your child is exaggerating the amount of pain he is in, you do need to take some counteraction. To your child, don't focus on how much pain he may or may not be in, but instead give reassurance that he will get better soon. Privately, though, think about the reasons this may be occurring. Your long-term strategy will be to try to focus on the causes.

Children, being the master manipulators that they are, will use their family's responses to their best advantage. Johnny, who bumped his head in the example above, may later complain of headaches or other pain to get some of the loving that he got with his accident. Sally might stay home from school for a day with a stomachache so Mom will stay with her and make her something nice to eat. These are normal and common responses in children, and they don't do any significant harm to anybody. However, what if Johnny or Sally stayed home for a week? Or a month? What if symptoms progressively worsened, garnering more and more attention? At some point a common behavior may evolve into a very harmful cycle, affecting the daily life of multiple family members and generating a great deal of concern or even medical tests. The increasing pain behaviors could occur both on a conscious level or an unconscious level.

Parents understandably have some conflicting feelings about their role when their child is in pain. On the one hand, they want to protect, nurture, and take care of their child. On the other hand, they also recognize the need to step back and encourage their child to push herself a little. In daily life, this conflict translates into the question: if my child has a headache, should I make her lie down? Should I make her go to school? Should I keep her from sports? Should I let her decide?

Overall, my advice is to stick as close to the daily routine as possible. For many children, school and other activities provide distractions that can help headaches go away. The very normalcy of sticking to the school routine often will decrease stress in many children, decreasing the amount of headaches and pain behavior. In regard to sports, if playing does not worsen the headache, then let your child participate if she feels up to it. (If playing sports does aggravate your child's condition, be sure to discuss this with your child's doctor.) Restricting your child's activities will increase stress, probably worsening rather than helping the headaches. In addition, your child may look for any twinge of a headache and exaggerate it, seeking evidence that activity is increasing his pain and trying to validate your concerns. Keep your child active rather than having her accept the role of "the sick one."

Don't worry: most parents actually do very well in evaluating and managing their child's pain! However, some parents may be giving their child cues that encourage pain behavior to grow.

Am I contributing to my child's pain behavior?

Ask yourself these questions:

- Do I respond to his complaints of pain emotionally? If so, could my emotional responses be encouraging more pain behavior?

- When he has a headache, do I encourage behavior associated with illness? Do I direct him to bed, give medicines, and promote other passive behaviors rather than encouraging him to continue his activities if possible?
- How do I feel about myself when I take care of my child? Emphasizing my nurturing qualities makes me feel good about myself, but can I nurture him in other ways instead?
- What other possible benefits do I get when my child feels sick? Do I get sympathy from others, time off from work, a sense of purpose in taking care of my child? Could I be transmitting the positive feedback that I may be getting to my child, which could have the effect of reinforcing his behavior?

Cultural Factors. Different cultures hold different views of pain, and this too can play a role in your child's experience. "Culture" includes not only your child's nationality, but also the influences he receives from books, movies, and people outside the family such as teachers and schoolmates. From all around, your child is receiving subtle or not-so-subtle cues about how to react and behave when she feels pain, and this starts very early on. Some of these cues will reinforce displays of pain, whereas others will discourage it.

Situational Factors. In different settings, a child may perceive different amounts of pain. For example, a headache that starts during playtime may not be "felt" as much as one that occurs in the midst of less pleasurable activities. Most parents are well aware of this, and become more concerned when the headaches their child experiences interrupts and takes the child from activities she normally enjoys. Using interruption of play to gauge if the headaches are worsening does make some sense, but it is not necessarily a cause for alarm.

A common example of a situation that exacerbates headaches is stress. Stressful situations are a well-known cause of headaches in many children. Exactly what physiologic changes occur in response to stress—which hormones increase, which parts of the brain are activated, what immune responses occur—are unclear, and therefore exactly how headaches are generated from stress is also unclear. Some children will react to a stressful situation by having a headache. This strategy may give your child a way to avoid dealing with the situation itself and may become a habitual response to stress if it is not recognized and dealt with. In other words, pain can become a way for a child to express—but not process—his emotions. In all likelihood, this will happen at an unconscious level. Your child may neither recognize that a situation is causing much stress for him nor recognize his body's response to it. You may be able to help him significantly by using biobehavioral treatment (see Chapter 5).

What other situational factors play a role in how much pain your child experiences? Looking at the research that has been done, one factor that seems to be important is whether or not the child feels in control. Settings in which the child feels helpless tend to produce more feelings of pain than when the child feels in command of the situation. For example, let's say that your child has to have blood drawn. Giving enough information about what will be happening, as well as giving him control over which arm the needle will go in, will result in feelings of participation and power. Despite the fact that the actual amount of pain will be the same, his anxiety and fear will be substantially diminished and he will have has a feeling of empowerment. The overall pain experience will be much less.

How do you give your child a feeling of control over a headache?

As stated previously, one way to diminish your child's pain is to give him a feeling of control. How do you do this when your child's headaches are largely unpredictable in when they happen?

Give your child as much information about the headaches as possible, so that he will be prepared when the headaches happen. Let him know that the headaches are not dangerous, and that they will be over soon. Remind your child that he has had headaches like this before, and he was OK then. For young children (of less than eight years) you may want to reinforce that the headaches are not happening as a punishment (remember, young children often see pain as punishment for breaking some rule). Make sure that your child understands that you are not worried. Children generally derive a lot of comfort from routines, especially at times when they are feeling anxious. Therefore, giving your child a consistent routine when he has a headache will also be helpful: "If you have a headache, first we will take some deep relaxing breaths, and if your headache is still there after a few minutes, we will lie down and maybe take medicine."

Give your child something that she can do, all by herself, to help the headaches go away. Younger children may try deep breathing exercises, or pressing on acupressure points, or simply telling somebody that she has a headache. Older children and teenagers can do all of those things, as well as deciding when to take medicine. Whatever the task, putting your child in charge of an aspect of the headaches will give her some degree of control over them. By focusing on the part that she can control, your child's anxiety and distress will be lessened, and her overall experience will be improved.

Look for factors your child can control in order to prevent headaches from happening. Keeping a headache diary may be a help, and this exercise is discussed more fully in Chapter 5 and Appendix A, but it may be that you and your child can already identify factors such as stress or certain foods that tend to trigger headaches. If you can, put your child in charge of avoiding those triggers. For example, if your child's headaches are triggered by caffeinated drinks, teach your child to order the correct beverages in the restaurant rather than ordering for him. If he goes ahead and has the caffeine anyway, then suffers the headache, remind him that the headache happened because he drank the soda. In a nonemotional way, remind him that the headache is a consequence of, rather than punishment for, his action. Your child will then clearly understand that he has control over at least some of his headaches, and he can make the choice of what he eats or drinks rather than having this become a control struggle for you.

Of course, headaches can vary a lot in terms of frequency, severity, and duration. These strategies may help only a little in your child's particular situation, and of course some children will respond to them better than others. Your child will likely need reinforcement of these messages over and over, until his responses become automatic and he can manage his headaches on his own. ("OK, the headache is starting, but it's no cause for concern. I'm going to relax first, then see if the headache is going away.") Give your child time to establish these strategies, offering lots of positive reinforcement when they work out and lots of understanding if they don't. You will be giving your child a powerful strategy to cope with pain.

Attitude. Assuming that you and your child's doctor have established that the headaches are not reflective of an underlying progressive problem like a brain tumor, you and your child should operate under the assumption that the headaches will get better. It is easy to get discouraged, especially if your child is having lots of headaches and has been on a lot of different medications. However, if *you* develop the attitude of "he's been through everything, and nothing is going to work," your child will think this, too, and this attitude will eventually become the reality. Children who have low expectations for their treatments will have lower response rates. The longer this goes on and the more treatments that have been tried, the more this attitude will build up.

Parents can add to a negative attitude in several ways. Watching their child in pain naturally makes parents anxious and upset, and they may not be patient enough to give the medications time to work. It may take the medication a couple of hours or so to start to get rid of the headache, and parents need to remind their children of this rather than say, "this one's not working either," after half an hour.

Parents who themselves had experienced headaches as children may think that since they suffered through childhood, their children will, too. If the parents continue to experience headaches as adults, they may see no way out for their children. This is especially true in the case of migraines, which are likely to be passed on through families. Parents may have been told that their child's headaches stem from genetic factors—that their children are prone to headaches because of inherited tendencies. Parents may then assume that because these headaches are "written into a child's genes," their child is destined to suffer from these headaches for the rest of his life. This is a wrong assumption. Your child can get better.

My child has been through so much because of his headaches. How can I have a positive attitude?

You have seen your child through a lot of headaches and have tried a lot of treatments, but nothing seems to work. How do you keep from being discouraged?

Remember some basics. Children have a wonderful rate of response to treatments, so if you haven't found what works for your child yet, you probably still will. Your child is always changing, growing, and maturing, and things will change for the better. The headaches likely did not develop overnight, and will not be cured overnight either.

Give treatments a chance. Give your child the prescribed medications, and be sure to administer the medicine exactly as directed by the child's doctor. For example, give the full dose instead of "under-dosing" because you fear possible side effects. Talk to your child's doctor about how long the medication may take to work, and then wait the full time to see if it does. Medications generally do not take pain away instantaneously, and many are measured in terms of their effectiveness after two hours. Some people who are taking a daily medication to prevent headaches may have to wait a month or two to see it work. Think about how you have evaluated medications in the past. Have you given them enough time to work?

Be realistic. Setbacks will happen. No treatment regimen will be 100 percent effective right away, and your child may develop a "breakthrough" headache at some point. Try not to interpret this headache as complete failure of the treatment regimen. Keeping a headache diary (see Chapter 5 and Appendix A) may help you keep your objectivity in evaluating the success of different treatments.

LESSONS TO BE LEARNED FROM THIS CHAPTER

In this chapter, we discussed different influences on your child's pain experience. The most important factor determining how your child experiences pain is his age. Other influences include the responses of parents and other family members, gender, cultural factors, personality factors, and the power of expectations.

Given all the factors discussed, what can you as a parent learn from them to best help your child through his headache experiences? Here are the major lessons to be learned:

- The experience of headache pain is not limited to unpleasant sensations generated by the body, but involves a complex mix of cognitive and emotional factors as well.

- Children will perceive and interpret their headaches differently, depending on their age. These developmental differences should be taken into account when talking about the headaches with children, because different factors need to be emphasized at different ages.
- It is important to talk with children about their headaches. The information that children get will help diminish their pain by diminishing their anxiety.
- It is also important to give children as much control as possible in dealing with their headaches. Even young children should be involved actively in their own treatment.
- Headaches may be triggered by stress and other situational factors, and part of the pain experience may involve emotional responses. Dealing with these aspects is a crucial part of headache and pain management.
- Parents need to be aware of many aspects of their own response to their child's pain and may need to modify their current reactions. In general, parents need to present positive, calm, and reassuring attitudes when their child has headaches.
- The goal of treatment is to maintain a normal daily life for the child, with as few changes in routine as possible.

CHAPTER 2

Doctor, Is It a Brain Tumor?

The Causes of Headaches in Children

Headaches are not all the same! There are more than three hundred medical causes of headache. While some of these conditions lead to nonspecific headaches without distinctive qualities, others have more particular patterns.

It is important to understand how one headache can feel different from another, because these differences are the clues to tell you and your child's doctor the cause of the headache. In turn, that will help you and your child's doctor decide what to do about it, and how much to worry. Here are some of the key features to look for:

1. *The location of the headache.* Does the head hurt all over? In the front? In the back? Is one side worse than another? Does the headache stay in the same place, or shift from one area to another?
2. *The severity of the headache.* Is your child having headaches that really cause him to be in agony, or are the headaches mild? Does he have to stop what he is doing and lie down? Do they keep him out of school or away from activities that he really wants to do? Of course, everyone reacts to pain differently, and your child's personality will play a role in his reaction.
3. *Exacerbating features of the headache.* What makes the headache feel worse? For some children, it will be light or

noise. For others, it will be body position (lying down or standing up, for example).

4. *The length of the headache.* Are these "easy" headaches that go away in a few minutes? Or headaches that last for days while you try everything to get rid of them?
5. *The usual time of day of the headache.* Are these "morning only" headaches, or can they happen at any time? What about an association with exercising? Is there a pattern in regard to eating, such as just before a meal or snack? Is there any particular relationship to stressful situations, such as school? (Some children only get headaches during the school week.)
6. *Associated features.* Headaches can have different types of associated symptoms, such as fever, vomiting, or vision changes.

Doctors will use the different headache features to try and identify the cause of the headache (this is discussed more fully in Chapter 6). The rest of this chapter talks about different causes of headaches and what the headaches associated with these causes usually feel like. Remember that although a lot of different causes of headaches are discussed in this chapter, the majority of children's headaches will fall into one of two categories: migraine headaches (discussed in Chapter 3) or tension-type headaches.

BRAIN TUMORS

Brain tumors in children are a relatively rare cause of headache. They affect approximately 1,500 children per year in the United States (as compared, for example, to the 15 percent of all children in the United States who experience migraines). However, the thought that their child might have a brain tumor is one of the most common fears when parents bring their child to the doctor. Once it is determined that the cause is not a tumor, many families feel that they can live quite nicely with the headaches.

First, a little basic anatomy. In children with brain tumors, the tumor has approximately a 70 percent chance of being located in the bottom part of the brain. When tumors grow in this area, they frequently compress a very important system in the brain called the ventricular system. The ventricles produce and circulate a fluid called cerebrospinal fluid (CSF). If this system is unable to circulate the CSF properly, the fluid pressure builds up (see Figure 1).

The consequences of this accumulating pressure, as you can imagine, can include headache pain. The headache is usually worse after the child has been lying down all night, without the aid of gravity to help drain the system. Therefore, the typical headache associated with a brain tumor happens in the early morning. For reasons that are not entirely clear, these headaches are often associated with vomiting.

In a typical brain tumor, which is a mass that is slowly growing, the headaches occur with more and more frequency and severity. Dizziness may be associated with brain tumors. Your child's doctor may also detect signs of increasing fluid pressure

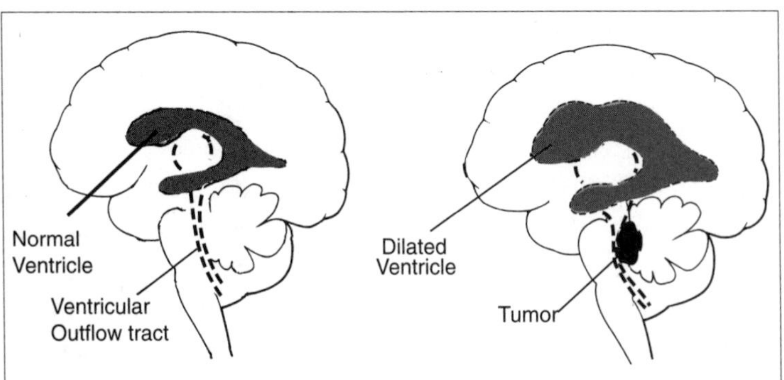

Figure 1. On the left, a normal brain. The ventricles are of normal size. On the right, a tumor compresses the outflow tract, causing the ventricles to enlarge.

on physical examination of your child, usually by looking in your child's eyes and checking his muscle tone and reflexes.

If your child's headaches typically occur in the morning and are associated with vomiting, be concerned but don't panic. Migraines, which are a far more common cause of headaches, also frequently occur in the morning and are also associated with throwing up.

Seizures are another symptom of brain tumors. Seizures are caused by abnormal bursts of electricity in the brain, and brain tumors, a focus of abnormal cells, often can be a starting point for the seizures. Seizures are usually caused by brain tumors located toward the surface of the brain, which is a more common location for tumors in older children and adults. However, if your child has seizures, again there is still a low chance of a brain tumor. Seizures occur in up to 5 percent of all children, whereas brain tumors are far less common (two to five occurrences per 100,000 children). Seizures are also, for reasons that are not clear, more frequent in patients with migraines.

Most doctors, if they think that a child is suffering from a benign headache disorder like migraines, will try to treat the headaches without getting a CT or MRI scan. The key for you and your child is remaining in contact with your child's doctor and letting him know if the prescribed treatment worked. If it didn't, your child's doctor will think about why it might not have worked, and at that point more tests might be done. In the process, a previously unsuspected tumor may be discovered. It's important to follow up and give your child's doctor the feedback.

Brain tumors, of course, can form in children who have previously been suffering from migraines or other types of headaches. If your child has a previous pattern of headaches that changes or worsens, it is important to let your doctor know of the change. If your child has suffered from headaches that have been stable for months, however, the likelihood of a tumor is quite small.

Example of a child whose headaches represent a brain tumor

Sally, a beautiful little girl who had just celebrated her fourth birthday, was having a difficult few weeks. She had been throwing up, especially in the morning, and first was thought to have some sort of a stomach bug. However, the nausea kept happening, and it got worse and worse. She would often awaken by throwing up repeatedly, and would then begin to cry. She "just didn't look so good," said her mother. Sometimes Sally would grab her head or say it hurt. She was falling more frequently than usual. Then a seizure occurred.

Sally's parents brought her to their pediatrician, who ordered an MRI scan. Done at the local hospital, the test required mild sedation. Unfortunately, the test revealed a brain tumor in the lower portion of the brain. Treatment was begun and Sally's symptoms began to improve.

TENSION-TYPE HEADACHES

Tension-type headaches (which used to be known as muscle contraction headaches) are one of the most common types of headaches. Tension-type headaches can be episodic (coming and going) or chronic (lasting for days or longer). Statistics in children are lacking, partly because the majority of children with tension-type headaches probably do not seek medical attention, and also because it can be hard to distinguish a tension-type headache from a migraine headache. Tension and migraine headaches, once thought to be dissimilar, are probably related in many ways.

It was previously thought that this type of headache pain was actually generated from contraction of muscles in the head or neck area. However, one reason the name was changed to tension-type headache was because it's unclear just how much of the pain is due to muscle contraction. There may be just as much contraction of head and neck muscles in migraine headaches as in tension-type headaches. We really do not know exactly why these headaches start, and why they can last for so long. In adults, biochemical changes in platelets (the cells in the blood that clot) are seen and certain chemicals found in the brain are thought to be affected, but the mechanism of how these changes might cause (or be caused by) headache is unclear. Different pain thresholds in different people could also play a role. Some people may be more sensitive to pain than others, and so may perceive certain physiologic changes as pain, whereas others would not be bothered by them.

Typically, a tension-type headache has a gradual onset over hours or days. The headache is usually on both sides of the head at once, and is usually either in the forehead/temple areas or the back of the head. These headaches are typically worse at the end of the school day or in the evening, and may last for days or longer. They are not typically associated with vomiting. They may be present over a period of years, without significant worsening.

The longer the headache goes on, the more likely it is to be associated with anxiety or depression. This is a real "chicken or egg" situation. Is the headache caused (or worsened) by the depression or anxiety, or are the abnormal moods caused (or worsened) by the headache? Clinical research does not give us a clear answer. This must be investigated on a patient-by-patient basis. Children today have a lot of stress in their lives, both in school and at home, and even the youngest children respond to tension around them. It is important to consider stress as a possible cause for these headaches, especially if another cause is not more evident.

Tension-type headaches can be treated in a variety of ways. Sometimes simple physical interventions can be quite effective, such as massage of the muscles in the head and neck areas. Warm moist heat in the form of a hot wet towel applied to the head and neck can also help. These interventions, which can be done at home by a parent, are aimed at relaxing both muscles and mind. More formal physical therapy can also be helpful. A physical therapist will help stretch and relax muscles through a variety of techniques, and can also help identify ways in which your child's body posture can be contributing to the headache. For example, these days children are carrying around very heavy textbooks and often laptop computers—all in one heavy backpack hanging off a shoulder. Unfortunately, informal or formal physical therapy has not been proven to be effective for very chronic forms of tension-type headache, but it may be helpful for less recalcitrant cases.

Other nondrug types of treatments can be effective, such as stress management or biofeedback. The general idea behind these therapies is for your child to learn to teach his body to relax (for a fuller discussion, see Chapter 5). These may take a while to work, but the lessons learned from these types of techniques are often helpful in dealing with life's stressors in general. Stress can affect many systems in the body, and teaching self-relaxation techniques is probably helpful in preventing not just headaches but other problems as well (such as stress-related stomach ulcers).

Medications can be effective. Anti-inflammatory medications such as aspirin and acetaminophen can be useful; ibuprofen and naproxen may be slightly more helpful. These can all be purchased without a prescription and are sold under various trade names (Advil, Motrin, Naprosyn, Tylenol). However, if taken every day or if taken more often than directed on the bottle, these medications can lead to "rebound" headaches in which the headaches become more frequent. For tension-type headaches that are happening frequently or are very severe, your child might benefit from a medication to be taken on a daily basis to prevent the headaches from occurring in the first place. How frequent is frequent and how severe is severe? It depends on the child, and how much the headaches are affecting his daily life. Taking a medication every day requires a careful assessment of the risk/benefit ratio for doing so (see Chapter 4 for a more complete discussion, and also for details of the different preventative medications that could be used). If your child is missing significant amounts of school, he should be on a preventative medication. There are a variety of preventative medications that may be prescribed. These include several categories of antidepressants as well as medications more traditionally used to prevent migraines (beta blockers, antiepileptics).

Example of a child with tension-type headaches

Katherine, a fifteen-year-old sophomore in high school, was fairly healthy. She had occasional headaches, but these were usually treated with acetaminophen or ibuprofen and would eventually go away. This fall, however, her headaches started to occur with increasing frequency. She described them as a dull ache all over her head, probably worse behind her eyes or at her temples (it was difficult for her to describe). She began to miss more and more school, first spending time in the nurse's office, then leaving school early, then missing whole days, and then hardly being there at all. She seemed to have a headache all the time. She began sleeping until one or two in the afternoon and staying up late. Her family was frustrated with her and wondered whether she was "faking it" and also wanted to know how to "snap her out of it." Katherine was frustrated with herself. She had previously done well in school, but now she might have to repeat the year. Feelings of depression and inadequacy began to grow, and the headaches got worse.

This situation, having progressed so far and having so many factors, could not be resolved immediately. It was hard to tell which was the bigger problem: the actual pain, or the behaviors surrounding it. Katherine was encouraged to make her life more normal: get up as if she were going to school, exercise regularly, eat regularly, and participate in school as much as possible—even if she didn't feel like it. She and her parents worked out a modified school program in which Katherine progressively worked back to a full schedule. Her parents and siblings were counseled that the combination of physical and psychological pain really made Katherine disabled from participating in her normal activities. It would be hard for anybody to judge how much "actual" pain was involved, and that probably wasn't the most important issue. The most important issue was getting Katherine back to full function. Her doctor recommended a combination of medications and cautioned Katherine against taking daily ibuprofen, as she had been doing. He also recommended a biofeedback program. Over the next two to three months, Katherine slowly improved and went back to school full time. She continued to have occasional headaches, but none that were quite so long-lasting and debilitating.

SINUS HEADACHES

The sinuses are hollow spaces in the head that are normally filled with air. The purpose of the sinuses is to produce and drain up to two pints of mucous every day. There are several different sinuses, each in different places in the head. The ones that most commonly cause headache are the paranasal sinuses: those located above the nose (in the forehead) and next to the nose (in the cheekbones). Sometimes, they can get infected or have fluid build up in them. This can generate intense pain because of the pressure of the fluid on the bony sides of the sinus cavities. Sometimes, this can be associated with fever as well. Usually, the pain is in the areas involved and may be described as "heavy." It usually starts out dull but can become throbbing. It will last for days or weeks. Pressing on the forehead and cheeks puts pressure on the sinuses directly underneath, and this can worsen the headache. Other factors that can make the pain worse are coughing and having the head down. Sufferers may also have a drippy nose, usually producing green or yellow mucous. Sometimes, especially in children, swelling of the eyelids can be seen. A cough sometimes occurs because of postnasal drip.

Children's sinuses are not well developed, and the younger the child, the less likely that sinus infections are the cause of the headaches. Special X rays or CT scans of the sinuses will really show whether sinuses are actually blocked. If the doctor is fairly certain that sinusitis is present, he may treat your child with a course of antibiotics without doing X rays or CT scans, however. The studies will probably be ordered if, after treatment, the child's headaches persist; at that point, knowing if the sinuses are blocked is extremely helpful.

Example of a child with sinus headaches

Jonah was only eight years old, but he had already been through a lot. His mother described him as "always sick, always with a cold, and always with a cold that lasts all winter." He had been on antibiotics off and on for most of his life, and almost continuously every winter. He always seemed congested. Allergists had diagnosed multiple allergies. ENT (ear, nose, and throat) specialists had done CT scans on his sinuses several times to document his sinus infections. In the past three years he had two operations to help his sinuses drain better. After each operation, he seemed to improve for a couple of months, but then he would go back to his normal stuffed-up state. Summers brought him relative relief. He participated on sports teams year-round with his friends, but he and his parents were tired of the constant problems with his nose.

Jonah had had more than his share of headaches, and his pediatrician finally referred him to a neurologist. Like the nasal congestion, the headaches seemed to be worse during the winter, but his parents had not really thought about whether his headaches worsened with flare-ups of his sinus problems. The headaches were fairly nondescript, with slowly worsening pain over both eyes and temples. His neurological exam was completely normal. Jonah's parents were sent home with instructions to keep a headache diary, recording when his headaches were worse and when his sinus problems were worse. They called back in December to confirm that it was pretty clear that both problems were flaring up together. His condition was treated with ibuprofen during the flare-ups, and he was sent back to the ENT doctor to see if anything else should be done to cure the baseline problem, the sinus infections.

EYESTRAIN HEADACHES

Eyestrain headaches refer to headaches that are caused by problems with nearsightedness in children. If a child is having difficulty seeing well, she will often scrunch up the muscles around her eyes in an effort to see better. Such muscle tensing can cause a headache, one that usually occurs when the child is trying to read a book or see the blackboard. The headache gradually fades when those activities are stopped. Fortunately, these headaches will improve with the right pair of corrective lenses!

This cause of headaches is thought to be more common than it probably is, but it is easy to check for with simple vision tests that can be done in a doctor's or optometrist's office. If the child is old enough, he will probably be able to tell you that he can't see the blackboard well, or perhaps his teacher will let you know. Many children are embarrassed about the possibility of needing glasses, and so may keep the information to themselves. However, you can look for a pattern of headaches that are worse during school or when the child has been looking at objects far away.

Except for refractive problems like nearsightedness, there are very few problems with the eyes themselves that will cause headaches. However, many types of headaches give patients pain in or behind the eye.

Example of a child with eyestrain headaches

Trevor, an eleven-year-old boy, used to love school, and he did very well in it. Then his grades began to slip. His parents noticed that he was not doing as much homework as he had the previous few months, but he did not think much of it until they talked with his teacher. His teacher told them that not only was Trevor not doing his homework half the time, but it was often wrong when he did do it. She wrote the assignments on the board the day they were assigned, and felt that it was the students' responsibility to copy down the assignment into their notebooks. She wondered if he had attention deficit problems, because he just seemed to be daydreaming all the time from his chair in the back of the room. Sometimes he would seem tired and put his head down.

Trevor was brought to his doctor's office to check out possible attention deficit disorder, and on a routine visual screening test it became apparent that his focusing problems were in his eyes, not his brain. His vision was about 20/100 in each eye. This was confirmed with an eye doctor's examination. When asked if he could see the assignments written on the blackboard, Trevor replied, "not really." When asked why he didn't tell anybody he was having difficulty, Trevor explained that he didn't want to wear glasses. He confirmed, though, that he thought his headaches were worse during school hours. Despite the subsequent problems that his parents had getting Trevor to actually wear his glasses, both grades and headaches improved rapidly after he got them.

DENTAL HEADACHES

The temporomandibular (TM) joint is the joint where the lower jaw (the mandible) attaches to the part of the skull near the temples (see Figure 2). Although the temporomandibular joint as a cause of headaches was first noted in the 1930s, very little attention was paid to this until recently. Problems in this joint, which can also cause problems in the way the teeth come together in a bite, can potentially lead to headaches. The joint can be affected by bruxism (grinding your teeth) and chronic gum chewing. Along with the actual joint, there is a large and very strong muscle (the masseter) involved. You can feel your masseter muscle by biting down and clenching your jaw; it bulges at the angle of your lower jaw. How often headaches arise from TM problems is both unclear and controversial; not all physicians agree that there is a relationship, especially in mild or moderate cases. Be very careful if somebody is telling you they can fix your child's headaches with surgery on their TM joint!

The pain can be dull or sharp, and usually occurs in both temples. It worsens with movements of the jaw or chewing, and the masseters or the joint itself may be tender. The pain can come and go depending on how much the joint is activated, but may be worse in the morning after a night of teeth-grinding.

Your child's dentist may be the one to let you know that this is a problem, so bring your child to the dentist regularly. Your dentist will check your child's bite and examine the teeth for signs of abnormal patterns of use, which could indicate a problem with the TM joint. Usually, treatment involves anti-inflammatory agents, massage or heat to the affected areas, and may also involve a "bite-block," a device worn at night that prevents teeth from grinding. However, there is not much in the way of formal proof that these strategies work. Certainly there are many people who have dental problems who don't get headaches.

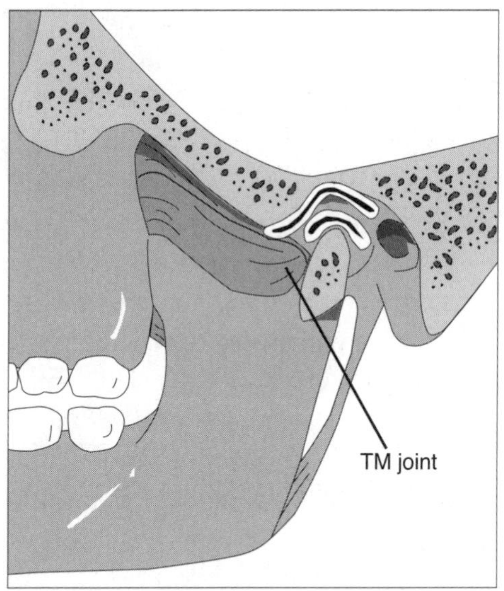

Figure 2. The temporomandibular (TM) joint.

Besides TM joint problems, infections in teeth can cause headaches. Children get tooth infections for many different reasons. Some children consume too much sugar, which predisposes them to cavities. In the very young (one- to three-year-olds, especially), children are often left to fall asleep at night with a bottle in their mouths to comfort them. This can cause many teeth to rot at once. Poor dental hygiene (insufficient brushing) is another way to get cavities. In any case, the pain can usually be localized to a particular tooth in the beginning, but as the infection spreads into the jaw (or up into nearby sinuses) it actually may not be as obvious. Diagnosis may involve X rays.

Example of a child with dental headaches

Seventeen-year-old Samantha, who had just completed final exams, developed frequent headaches, especially in the morning. They were not particularly severe and usually went away on their own, but they were happening frequently. Samantha thought about going to her primary care physician to talk about them, but when she went for her regular dental checkup, her dentist noticed that her teeth were looking worn down in several areas. He fitted her with a bite block, and her headaches improved.

MENINGITIS

The meninges are special membranes that cover the brain and spinal cord. They wrap around these organs, extending from the head down through the neck and spinal column. Their function includes protection and nourishment of the central nervous system.

The meninges can get infected by certain viruses, bacteria, and fungi, which can all invade this area. The infection can easily spread throughout the space between the brain and the meninges; as this progresses, pressure can build up on the brain, or the infectious agents themselves can infect the brain as well. As one can imagine, this causes a person to become very ill. You "catch" meningitis just like you "catch" a cold; fortunately, it is much more rare. Bacterial meningitis is seen in approximately five to ten cases per 100,000 people per year. Even if properly treated, the mortality rate (the percentage of people who have the disease who die) is about 10 percent.

Bacterial meningitis needs to be rapidly diagnosed and treated; otherwise it can be fatal quite rapidly. The onset of the headache is typically rapid, worsening over a few hours. The pain can be anywhere in the head, but a fairly characteristic feature of the pain is a stiff neck, where it is quite painful to bend the head forward. Some types of bacterial meningitis are associated with a rash. People affected with bacterial meningitis will usually also have other symptoms such as sleepiness, vomiting, or seizures. They may also have sensitivity to light and sound, similar to migraines. The process will become progressive, leading to coma and death. The doctor can diagnose this type of problem with a CT scan and lumbar puncture. (A lumbar puncture is a procedure in which a sample of the fluid that bathes the brain and spinal cord is removed and sent for laboratory analysis; see Chapter 6 for details.) Antibiotics should be started intravenously immediately.

Viral meningitis is generally not as severe as bacterial meningitis. In fact, some people who have viral meningitis may not even know it. Most, however, suffer a week or so with a very bad headache, worse than any they have ever had. This condition is much more common than bacterial meningitis, and of all the "serious" causes of severe headaches, one of the most frequent.

Example of a child with meningitis

Three-year-old Justin had gone to bed the night before "a little cranky," said his parents. This was unusual for him; he was generally a chubby little angel. His forehead felt warm, but not too warm, and his parents thought he was developing a cold. However, when they woke him up the next morning, he was clearly quite sick. He had a red rash all over his body, a high fever, and every time they moved him he groaned. He did not talk but just clutched at his blanket, and didn't want to wake up. He looked so ill his parents brought him to the emergency room. The nurse looked at him, took his temperature and vital signs, and came back quickly with the doctor. The doctor ordered a CT scan immediately, and as the scan was finishing up Justin had a seizure. They raced him back to the emergency room, where they drew blood and did a lumbar puncture. Justin, quite sleepy after his seizure, barely moved as they positioned him, inserted a needle in his back, and withdrew fluid. The fluid appeared cloudy. Justin was started on antibiotics as well as antiseizure medications, and he was admitted to the intensive care unit.

In the unit, Justin remained quite sleepy over the next day or so but then began to improve. He did not have any further seizures. He was given ten days of intravenous antibiotics, and by the time they were done he was his usual happy self.

BLEEDING

Blood vessels in the head can break open from a variety of causes. This can lead to very severe headaches. Above and beyond the pain, however, bleeding in the head is dangerous, frequently immediately life-threatening. There is only a fixed volume that can be held inside the skull; if the volume of blood starts to increase because of bleeding, the volume of the brain will become compressed and damaged. This is very dangerous and generally leads to disability or death.

Bleeding can happen in several different areas, depending on the cause. One place bleeding can occur is between the skull and the outer lining of the brain (the outer lining is a tough membrane called the dura mater). This type of bleeding is called epidural (meaning "outside the dura") bleeding. One common cause of this type of bleeding is a blow to the head, such as a baseball bat striking the temple or trauma from an auto accident. A break in the bones of the skull does not need to occur. The trauma of the impact can injure certain blood vessels, which can then bleed quite rapidly. This would usually cause a mild to moderate headache followed by loss of consciousness. There may also be weakness on one side of the body and/or an enlarging and unreactive pupil in one eye. Depending on how rapidly the bleeding occurs, the progression of symptoms could be faster or slower. Usually emergency surgery is required to drain the blood that has accumulated and stop the bleeding. However, occasionally with slower bleeds, they will stop on their own.

Another place bleeding can occur is just under the same covering of the brain (subdural). The most common way this occurs is when the head is struck by a hard object that does not penetrate the skull. The bleeding can happen quickly or more slowly, so again there can be rapid or gradual worsening of symptoms. Symptoms usually consist of increasing sleepiness, personality changes or changes in the ability to think, and may again include a mild to moderate headache, weakness on one side of the body, and/or an enlarging and unreactive pupil. However, subdural bleeding can progress quite slowly and reach a large size without many symptoms. Headache is one of the most common symptoms, but it can be fluctuating. The headache is usually on the sides of the head.

A third way bleeding can occur is from the rupture of a blood vessel surrounding or inside the brain itself. An aneurysm is a weakening of the wall of a blood vessel; over time, it will pouch out and may break open. This is an extremely rare event in children, but a family history of brain aneurysms increases the likelihood of a child having an aneurysm. More frequent in children are abnormally formed tangles of blood vessels called arteriovenous malformations (AVMs), which can also bleed. The headaches associated with these problems are typically explosive, described as a "thunderclap" by those who survive. It is characteristically overwhelmingly severe from the onset, and frequently patients will lose consciousness very quickly. Vomiting is often associated with the condition and makes the pain worse. A diagnosis needs to be made quickly, and because of the severity of the symptoms would nearly always be done in a hospital emergency room. Treatment may include surgery.

Bleeding of smaller vessels within the brain can also occur. This will often cause a headache in association with the physical symptoms of a stroke. The symptoms will vary depending on what part of the brain is involved but could include weakness of an arm and/or a leg. The headache often starts out on the same side of the head as the bleeding but may involve the whole head. If the bleeding happens in the back or lower portion of the brain, the headache is also in the back of the head. This location is fairly dangerous, as bleeding there can rapidly compress vital parts of the brain. Bleeding in this area is often associated with vomiting and unconsciousness. Emergency surgery is often required.

Example of a child with an intracranial bleed

Fifteen-year-old Alex was in church with his family, and everything seemed to be fine. All of a sudden he stood up with a loud groan and tried to walk to the back of the church. His mother noticed that he was quite pale, sweaty, and was grabbing the back of his head. He stumbled and fell to the floor. An ambulance was called.

At the hospital, an emergency CT scan showed bleeding on the left side of his head. A procedure called an angiogram was done, which showed a tangle of abnormally formed vessels that caused the bleed. A clip was placed on the vessels in a surgical procedure. Alex woke up the next day with a fairly severe headache, but that improved over the next few days. He also had some mild right-sided weakness. After awhile, that improved to the point where it was hardly noticeable.

POST-TRAUMATIC HEADACHES

These types of headaches—headaches that develop after injuries—are very common. A child who has been in an accident may develop headaches shortly after the accident, and sometimes these take a long time to go away. The accident may not involve direct forceful contact to the head. So, for example, a child could have headaches triggered when he is in an automobile accident, even if his head did not directly hit anything during the accident.

These headaches can be quite frightening to parents for several reasons. For one thing, scattered stories are carried in the general news about children who have major medical problems or even die after seemingly minor head injuries. For another, after an accident you can't just inspect the brain or the area around it for bleeding; unlike other body parts, you won't see bruising or swelling. Finally, post-traumatic headaches are frequently accompanied by other problems that can be alarming, such as increased sleepiness, difficulty thinking, or emotional changes. When these problems are involved the child will usually be diagnosed as having a post-traumatic syndrome or a post-concussive syndrome.

These headaches can be of several types. Some can be associated with neck pain. Some can seem more like migraines; others may seem more like tension-type. If the headaches are associated with sleepiness or difficulty thinking, a CT scan to look for any bleeding problems is in order, especially if symptoms are worsening. Sometimes seizures can be generated by the brain injury, and some doctors may order an EEG (electroencephalogram) to look for them, depending on your child's symptoms.

These headaches can persist for a long time and can be difficult to manage. One study showed that even a year after experiencing the head trauma, up to about a third of people will continue to have headaches. Treatment will often depend on the particular symptoms of the headache (for example, using migraine drugs for some of the headaches that have migraine-like qualities). Depending on how frequently the headaches occur, your doctor might prescribe medications or biofeedback as part of a preventative strategy. But some of the medications may worsen some of the symptoms of the post-traumatic syndrome, such as making the child sleepier. Occasionally the headaches will be so severe that the child will need to cut back on school or other obligations, but this should only be done in severe cases. Since these headaches can go on for a long time, the message to the child should be: keep functioning, even if you have a headache.

Example of a child with post-traumatic headaches

Brian used to be an "A" student at school. In his spare time, he enjoyed rollerblading. One Friday evening shortly after his fifteenth birthday, he went skating down the slight hill of his driveway, which he had done hundreds of times before. That's the last thing he remembered. He was found by a neighbor approximately ten minutes later, lying on his side (which was now quite bruised). He had not been wearing a helmet, and he was quite groggy. When his neighbor helped him to a seated position, Brian threw up. The neighbor noticed that his speech was a little slurred, but Brian was able to recognize him and, with help, get back to his parents' house. He was brought to the local emergency room.

There, a CT scan of his head was normal. No broken bones or internal injuries were found, and when Brian became more awake and was able to hold a conversation, he was released home. It was thought that he had been the victim of a hit-and-run accident by a car.

He took it fairly easy that weekend, lying on the couch, as he had some nagging headaches. They weren't severe, just persistent, and he and his parents felt that they would go away in time. However, when Monday came and Brian went to school, he was tired, felt that he "couldn't think straight," and had a headache; he left early and then took Tuesday and Wednesday off. When he didn't make it through school on Thursday or Friday, his parents became concerned and brought him to his pediatrician. His pediatrician advised them to try Tylenol as needed, and expected that things would improve over the next few weeks. However, a month later Brian still could not make it through a day of school, and he was referred to a neurologist.

The neurologist ran some tests measuring how well Brian could think and remember. His neurological exam was normal, with the exception of some difficulty with short-term memory. Brian was eventually placed on a daily medication to prevent headaches. Although he was initially even worse because the medication made him tired, the frequency of his headaches improved over the next two weeks. For breakthrough headaches, he was given a specific anti-migraine medication that helped. Brian's parents met with the school psychologist, and he was given a schedule which eased him back into a full school day over three weeks; meanwhile, he was expected to complete homework assignments at home. Although he continued to suffer headaches off and on for the next two years, he was able to function and complete high school. By the time he went to college he was back to normal.

STRESS

Dealing with the combined subjects of stress and headaches is difficult, because they are two invisible problems. For both, there is no objective evidence of what is occurring—there is no clear measure of how much stress or pain a person is experiencing. What is stressful or painful for one person may not bother another in the least; it is hard, then, for one person to understand exactly what the other is going through. This is often even more difficult when a parent who does not experience headaches or feel particularly stressed-out tries to understand a child who may be affected by headaches and stress. A parent who is full of tension and worry (about the spouse, the bills, the extended family, the kids—whatever it is) may look at her child and think—what does he have to worry about? He's got it easy!

But everyone worries. Kids tend to have different concerns than parents. The fears and worries of preschool children are familiar: they are afraid of the dark, worried that they might get owies, fearful that an out-of-sight parent might be gone forever. Younger school-age children (five to eight years) are dealing with both a whole new social situation and all new academic expectations at school. As children mature, they are dealing with increasingly difficult schoolwork, higher expectations regarding their own behavior, and complicated issues with their peers. Older adolescents are dealing with their rapidly changing bodies (and the intense hormonally-provoked feelings that go along with them), dating, school performance pressures ("These grades count for college"), and trying to fit in their newfound sense of independence with their old roles in the family unit. Throughout, children may be dealing with a variety of family disruptions: parents living in poverty, parents fighting or divorcing, the breakup of their family unit, or half-siblings coming in and out of the home in shared custody arrangements.

In addition, "down time," or time where children can relax and work out their stresses naturally, is fast disappearing. Articles about over-scheduled children have appeared throughout the popular press. It is not uncommon for even young school-age children to be involved in several extra-curricular activities. The increase in working parents has led to a rise of at-school daycare, so in many cases children are not even home until dinnertime.

Medically, we know that stress affects the body in a variety of ways, most of them bad. People under chronic stress may suffer more infectious illnesses, have more stomachaches and headaches, and have muscle spasms all over the body. However, the exact mechanisms behind this have not been thoroughly studied, as this is a relatively new field. Western medicine has been slow to acknowledge the effects of stress on the body.

Is your child stressed out?

Every child will respond to stressors in his or her own way. Some will withdraw, and some will become hyperactive. Some will be able to easily explain what is bothering them; others require weeks or months of working with a trained therapist.

Older children may escape to drugs, boyfriends, or girlfriends. How do you, as a parent, evaluate your child's stress level?

Know your child. This is absolutely the most important point. Communicate with your child and know what is going on in his life, throughout his life. You will not only be able to better understand his feelings, but your child, knowing you understand, will better be able to share his feelings.

Is your child a natural worrier? Some children have expressed worry or have had environmental sensitivities since the moment they could talk (or scream). These children may have been quite fussy as babies, paying more attention to (and being more bothered by) a variety of external and internal stimuli. Other children seem to have more "inner harmony" and don't seem to worry as much about things going on around them. In evaluating your child's level of worry, you need to take into account his baseline personality tendencies.

Look for changes in behavior. Is your once outgoing, happy child withdrawn or angry? Is your calm preschooler now a frenetic second-grader? Are there any changes in mood such as sudden, frequent crying or wild mood swings? Look for any reasons that may be behind the change and explore them in depth.

Does your child seem quite prone to illnesses? Although there could be many reasons behind this, stress is probably underestimated as a cause. Headaches and stomachaches are thought to be among the most common stress-related complaints (both, possibly, because of their abstract nature).

Has sleep been affected? Some children are naturally good sleepers; others have difficulty making it through a single night without waking up once or more. However, the tendency toward being a good or bad sleeper is fairly stable for a single child—it is unusual for a good sleeper to suddenly become a bad sleeper, for example. Rule out possible medical causes with your child's doctor (such as obstructive sleep apnea or seizures), but consider stress as a cause.

Has appetite been affected? Appetite can go either down or up with stress, with resulting weight loss or gain. Try to be alert before major changes occur.

Has schoolwork been affected? Usually stress is manifested by a drop in grades or truancy, but some children will pour energy into their schoolwork to escape stress in other aspects of their lives, or in the hope that they will attract notice and praise by an otherwise unsupportive parent. If your child is using drugs to escape daily stresses, grades are likely to drop (but do not always do so).

What can you as a parent do to help alleviate your child's stress? Remember the three As:

- Acknowledge. Don't deny that stress could be a possible problem for your child.
- Ask around. Get a fresh perspective from your child's friends, teachers, and other people who know your child as to what may be going on.
- Access help. There is help for your child both in the medical field as well as through a number of social services programs. Your child's pediatrician or family practice doctor will often be a good place to start; alternatively, talk to the principal or psychologist at your child's school.

ENVIRONMENTAL CAUSES OF HEADACHES

We are exposed to hundreds of thousands of chemicals, both natural and manmade, every day, via all of our senses. We breathe them in the form of perfumes, deodorizers, pollens, and smoke. We touch them in the form of household cleaners, personal hygiene products, plants, and animal products. We taste them in our food and drink. We are exposed to loud noises and bright lights. Could some of them be causing headaches?

The answer to this question is clearly yes, that some children's headaches are triggered by certain exposures. However, figuring out which children are affected is less clear. There is no way that a parent can keep track of every chemical to which a child is exposed, and even if that were possible, avoiding certain exposures may be difficult. Furthermore, whether a child has an environmental trigger is quite individual; some children will be affected while others, exposed to the same situations, will not.

One of the most common environmental triggers is loud noises. For children, this commonly occurs in the settings of parties and other places of excitement, and so sometimes sorting out whether the trigger is the noise or the other stimulation is quite difficult. Probably the easiest way to determine this would be to simply ask your child which part of the situation bothered him the most; some can answer quite specifically. After the headache starts, loud noises can also make it worse and the child should avoid loud noises as much as possible (a situation called phonophobia).

Another common trigger is bright lights, or other types of lighting situations. One of my patients found that being in rooms lighted with fluorescent lights seemed to trigger her headaches. Several parents have noted that bright sunny days can be hard on their kids, especially when the sun makes patterns through moving car windows. (Although most children living in the Seattle area, where I live, are so happy to see the sun that the headaches don't matter so much. My favorite joke about this area is about our numerous rainy days: "Little boy, does it ever stop raining here?" a stranger asks. "How should I know," the boy answers, "I'm only six!")

Cigarette smoke is truly an avoidable environmental trigger of headaches. Children who smoke (usually smoking begins in adolescents, but of course it can start earlier) or who are exposed to secondhand smoke are being exposed to a very potent headache stimulator. Cigarettes, of course, have nicotine in them to various degrees, but they also have a number of other chemicals in them that most people do not take into consideration.

One such chemical is carbon monoxide. Both nicotine and carbon monoxide have effects on cerebral blood vessels, the nicotine constricting them and the carbon monoxide relaxing them; it may be that the interplay causes headaches through this mechanism. Carbon monoxide, in and of itself, can cause headaches thought to result from its irreversible binding of oxygen in the blood stream (making the oxygen less available to brain cells). We are finding out that secondhand smoke may be at least as dangerous as smoking itself to some children. If one of my chronic headache patients is a smoker or exposed to secondhand smoke, usually my first recommendation is to stop the exposure and see if the headaches improve on their own.

Does mercury cause headaches?

Several years ago, the television show *60 Minutes* broadcast a story about the possible dangers of mercury dental fillings. This brought to national attention a controversy about whether these types of fillings are dangerous, and headaches have been listed as one of the potential dangers. Certainly, some dentists prefer not to use mercury fillings because of the potential danger, although most dentists do feel that it is safe. There really is not a lot of evidence to the contrary. Some people who have had mercury fillings placed and then suffered from headaches have had them removed; there are no good statistics about the results, however. Also, this is a situation that generally affects adults (who are more likely to have such fillings). One patient that I have treated had his mercury fillings removed, with no noticeable improvement.

However, there has been recent evidence that some fish from polluted waters contain mercury at levels high enough to pose a possible health threat. These fish may cause a variety of neurologic problems including headache. Further study is needed.

HEADACHES FROM FOOD

Do certain foods give children headaches? The relationship between migraines and particular foods has been studied much more thoroughly in adults than in children. Some adults find that eating a particular food or drinking a particular drink will lead to headaches, and by avoiding those foods or drinks, they will prevent most or all of their headaches from occurring in the first place.

Examples of foods that commonly trigger migraines in adults include yellow cheeses like cheddar, red wine, and food containing monosodium glutamate (MSG), a common flavor additive. Other common examples include nitrates (a meat preservative plentiful in hot dogs) and aspartame (brand names NutraSweet and Equal). However, so many products have been linked to headaches that one couldn't possibly cut all of them out in the hopes of eliminating headaches—a more individualized approach is necessary. Products that trigger headaches in some people are well tolerated in others. In contrast, foods that are seemingly unobjectionable to most people will be difficult for others to tolerate (one of my patient's most potent triggers was whole wheat bread).

Certainly some foods can trigger headaches in some children on a regular basis. However, I find that the relationship in general is less predictable than with adults. A thirteen-year-old patient of mine, Max, once told me that one particular brand of root beer spelled trouble for him, but he could drink every other kind of root beer without a problem (and it was unrelated to the caffeine content of the drink). Another patient, sixteen-year-old Jenna, who suffered from migraines for years, found that foods (or medications) containing a particular red dye triggered her headaches. Many parents are familiar with headaches in children following birthday parties, and refined sugar has frequently been identified as a culprit. (However, especially in the case of birthday parties, so much stimulation is around that it's hard to be sure what is causing the problems!)

Overall, our diets contain more and more processed foods, man-made chemicals, and sugar than ever before. One study estimated that our diet contains exposure to some ten thousand chemical additives in the form of artificial flavoring and coloring, preservatives, thickeners, antibacterial agents, and even hormones. Salt consumption is increasing: a 1994 survey showed that Americans are eating twenty-two pounds of salty snacks per year compared to seventeen-and-a-half pounds in 1977. (Some people swear that salt gives them headaches; others profess that salt takes them away.) Children ages five to sixteen drank 23 percent more soft drinks than in 1977—soft drinks that have no nutritional value but expose children to all sorts of manufactured chemicals and large amounts of sugar and artificial sweeteners. The consumption of soft drinks is increasing further, especially in schools. This fact was illustrated by a 1999 National Public Radio story detailing the relationship between schools and soft drink manufacturers. The manufacturers are providing schools with a great deal of money in exchange for soft drink machines being placed all over campus, in addition to other types of advertisement in the school itself.

Let's even take the case of a simple, natural product like sugar. The amount of sugar we are consuming is increasing at an astounding rate. Americans right now consume almost 30 percent more sugar than we did in 1970, and that rate is expected to increase by 16 percent over the next ten years. The USDA recommends consuming no more than twelve teaspoons (forty-eight grams) daily for adults, but the average American takes in four times as much. Part of the reason is that food companies have been raising the sugar content of their products, as well as increasing the number of sweetened products they prepare. The more sugar we eat, the more we want to eat—a non-sweetened diet tastes quite bland after our tastebuds become accustomed to a sugary menu. We buy more sweetened products, and the cycle perpetuates itself. The situation is even worse for children; whereas adults like the taste of sugar-containing foods only when the sugar content is kept under 12 percent (after that it is perceived as too sweet), children love foods where the sugar content exceeds even 20 percent. So food targeted to children gets loaded up with a substance that has no nutritional value whatsoever. Furthermore, they will carry these tastes with them into and throughout adulthood.

So where do you start when you are trying to figure out if your child's food intake is causing his headaches? The first step is to establish whether there is a relationship between any particular food your child eats and when his headaches occur. This can be best done with the use of a headache diary. (See Chapter 5 for tips on establishing a headache diary, and Appendix A for a sample diary.) If a relationship is seen, that may be a trigger for your child's headaches. Try cutting out the food to see if the headaches will go away.

What is hypoglycemia? Can it be causing my child's headaches?

Hypoglycemia refers to a concentration of blood sugar that is too low. The concentration of sugar in your blood is determined by a variety of factors, but mainly by achieving a balance between two major hormones, insulin and glucagon. Insulin lowers your blood sugar, and glucagon raises it. Diabetics have high blood sugar levels because of low insulin levels and need to take insulin as a medication to control their blood sugar. When they are given too much insulin, their blood sugar may drop too low and they may get headaches, clamminess, and shakiness as some of the initial symptoms; if their blood sugar drops further they may lose consciousness or suffer brain damage. This type of hypoglycemia has clearly been documented.

What is more controversial is whether hypoglycemia accounts for a variety of symptoms—headaches, bad moods, paleness of skin, to name a few—in nondiabetic, otherwise healthy people of all ages. Many people list themselves or their children as being hypoglycemic because they get hungry easily and, prior to eating, may experience the above symptoms. However, the vast majority of these people have not had their blood sugar measured and would not qualify for a medical diagnosis of hypoglycemia. Of those who do have their blood sugar checked, many will not be able to show that their symptoms correlate with low blood sugar levels.

Whether we can identify the exact trigger for these symptoms—low blood sugar or other metabolic changes—it is clear that some people are more sensitive to eating patterns than others. Some people do well on two or three meals a day, others need a more constant influx of food to prevent headaches or other symptoms from occurring. Children with migraines may be especially sensitive to hunger or thirst; pay attention to when your child typically has headaches in relationship to when he eats.

MENSTRUAL MIGRAINES

It's no surprise to most women to find that menstruation is a frequent trigger of headaches. Migraines in particular tend to be provoked by menstruation. For some women, this is the only time they get headaches. Most of the time, headaches occur right around menstruation, a time when estrogen levels fluctuate greatly.

Adolescent girls are more likely to have their migraines start at about the time of puberty. Their headaches may develop a cyclical pattern in the year or so before menstruation actually begins. In all likelihood this reflects underlying hormonal changes.

Preventative treatment can include medications given right around the time of the period to try to prevent the headaches from occurring. Magnesium supplementation has been helpful for some. In addition, standard treatments for stopping headaches once they start can be used for relief.

MIGRAINES AND ORAL CONTRACEPTIVES ("THE PILL")

What if your adolescent daughter with migraines wants to be on oral contraceptives? What if your doctor is suggesting oral contraceptives as a way to treat your daughter's migraines?

In some girls, being put on oral contraceptives will provoke headaches or make an existing headache disorder worse. In others, being put on them will make headaches better. "The Pill," therefore, is both a cause of and a treatment for headaches, most of which are thought to be migraines. It is difficult to predict who will be affected in which way, but if your daughter had headaches start after she has been on oral contraceptives, remember that that could be a trigger. Some are affected the very first cycle; others may be affected after longer use. If oral contraceptives are identified as a possible trigger and are to be stopped, it may take several menstrual cycles for the headaches to go away.

The amount of estrogen in the pills may be a factor in how headache-provoking they are. Switching to low-estrogen or progesterone-only varieties may be of help.

There is also controversy about whether oral contraceptives increase the risk of stroke in people with migraine headaches. Some studies have shown this to be the case, but most of these were done with higher-dose estrogen pills than most people use now (and the women studied were generally not adolescents). If there is a prominent history of stroke in your family, and if your daughter has migraines (and especially if she smokes, another risk factor for both stroke and migraine), discuss the risks and benefits of oral contraceptives with her doctor. Remember, though, that pregnancy also carries significant risks!

REBOUND HEADACHES

A number of children who have daily headaches may have them, paradoxically, because of the medications they are taking to control them. At least in adults (there is no such statistical information available for the pediatric population) 80 percent of daily headaches may be medication-related, or "rebound" headaches.

Usually children are started on a medication by their physician (or parents start them on an over-the-counter medication) for pain relief from their headaches. The medication works great. They use the medication frequently for relief of their pain. It still works great, but their headache frequency begins to accelerate. They use the medication more. It still does the trick, but maybe takes a little longer to work and relief may not last as long as it used to; the headache comes back again sooner. Soon children are having headaches every day and taking medications for them every day, and are generally unhappy and frustrated with the whole situation.

These types of headaches can be quite variable, from a dull ache all over the head to a throbbing, pulsating migraine. Frequently, they can last so long that they are virtually constant, and as one can imagine, this can turn into a depressing and energy-depleting situation for the headache sufferer.

What medications can cause rebound headaches? One thing that surprises most people is that medications bought over the counter, perceived as "not very strong," are among the most frequent culprits. Be especially wary of medications that contain caffeine in them (caffeine, in and of itself, can also cause rebound headaches; see the section "Headaches From Food," page 56).

Here are the most common culprits:

- Any over-the-counter pain relievers (aspirin, ibuprofen, acetaminophen, naproxen), especially those that also contain caffeine (such as Excedrin Migraine)

- The "triptan" migraine medications: sumatriptan (Imitrex), rizatriptan (Maxalt), naratriptan (Amerge), zolmitriptan (Zomig), etc.
- Barbiturates or medications which contain them (Fiorinal, Fioricet, Esgic)
- Narcotics (Tylenol with codeine, Demerol, Vicodin, Percocet)
- Ergotamines (Cafergot, Wigraine)

Opinions vary as to the exact method that would best stop the cycle. Some advocate a "cold turkey" method, in which the offending substance is stopped all at once. Your child, in this case, may get a fairly severe withdrawal headache within twenty-four hours of stopping the offending medication; however, after that he may not have any further headaches from it. Others advocate a slower withdrawal process, cutting the medication back gradually. The resulting withdrawal headaches may be milder, but more numerous. In either case, don't treat the withdrawal headache with the medication you are trying to cut back on!

The trick with rebound headaches, of course, is diagnosing them. How can you tell if the headache is from too much medication, or whether the baseline headache disorder is getting worse? Since rebound headaches are not a distinctive type, you can't really tell for sure without actually withdrawing the medication and seeing whether the headaches improve. Rebound headaches should not be associated with troublesome features like seizures, vomiting, weakness, numbness, or other worrisome signs, especially if those signs are new. If those signs appear, one would have to suspect a worsening of the baseline headache disorder—and steps should be taken to find out why. However, if those signs don't appear, then stopping (or severely limiting) the above medications is an important next step. These medications were not designed to be taken on a daily or near-daily basis; who knows what all of the potential side effects of doing so really are?

IDIOPATHIC INTRACRANIAL HYPERTENSION (IIH)

Idiopathic intracranial hypertension (IIH) is an important cause of headache in children because although it is rare, it can have severe consequences. Older names include *pseudotumor cerebri* or *benign intra-cranial hypertension,* but the condition has nothing to do with brain tumors of any sort. IIH is a condition in which the cerebrospinal fluid (CSF) that circulates within the chambers of the brain is at too high a pressure. The first word in the name, *idiopathic,* means that nobody really knows why it occurs. It probably happens for a variety of reasons, as it is associated with a number of different medical conditions. It may be slightly more likely to affect girls than boys. IIH can be associated with endocrine problems such as thyroid problems, abnormalities in the naturally produced steroids of the body, or growth hormone abnormalities. It is sometimes tied to certain medications such as phenytoin (a seizure medication), steroids, tetracycline antibiotics, and other medications. People with certain medical conditions are at higher risk, such as those with anemia, lupus, and kidney problems. Obesity is another risk factor. However, IIH can also occur in otherwise healthy children.

The major problem is that IIH will lead to permanent visual problems if left undiagnosed and untreated. That is why a previous name for the condition, *benign intracranial hypertension,* was inappropriate, as this is obviously not "benign" at all: vision loss is a serious consequence.

Nearly all patients who have this condition will have headaches. These headaches are nonspecific. They are usually all over the head, but can be felt in one part more than another; again, nobody really knows why this is the case. Vision can sometimes briefly cloud with these episodes. Sometimes, children will have double vision or other visual problems. Hearing "whooshing" sounds has been reported. Some children may throw up with these headaches.

The doctor who examines a child with this condition will almost always find a physical abnormality called papilledema. Papilledema refers to swelling of the optic nerve. The optic nerve can be seen as it enters the back of the eye; your doctor will examine your child by looking in his eyes with a tool called an ophthalmoscope (it's a specially magnified light source; see Chapter 6 for fuller discussion). Other signs might include restrictions or abnormalities of eye movements.

Treatment usually involves diuretics, with the idea being to reduce the pressure of the (CSF) as much as possible. If the child is overweight, weight loss is usually recommended. If the child does well, hopefully he could be weaned off the diuretics, but if he continues to have problems surgical procedures may need to be done (these include either installing a permanent shunt to divert fluid out of the system or cutting the sheaths around the optic nerves to prevent pressure from building up on them). In any case, the child will need to be followed by an eye doctor to make sure that vision remains intact.

Example of a child with idiopathic intracranial hypertension (IIH)

Although only fourteen years old, Angela already weighed more than two hundred pounds. She began to develop gradual headaches that worsened over a few months. When her eyes started to blur, her mother took her to the eye doctor, thinking that getting new glasses would probably help the headaches. Angela told the eye doctor that at times she felt as though her eyes were crossed and that she sometimes saw double. On exam, the doctor found that Angela's eyes were slightly out of alignment with each other and that she also had mild papilledema. An MRI was done (it came back as normal), and she was sent to a neurologist.

The neurologist performed a lumbar puncture in the office, during which a needle was inserted into Angela's back to measure the pressure of the fluid within (see Chapter 6 for further details of the procedure). The fluid went up into a tube called a manometer, which measured the pressure—and kept going up and up into the extension tubing. All in all, the pressure was at least twice as high as it should have been. Angela's headache immediately improved when the excess fluid was removed.

Angela was placed on diuretics and given a restricted diet, and her headaches significantly improved. Her eye doctor gave her another exam and determined that she had normal vision. After a few months, her doctor tried to take her off the diuretics, but her headaches returned shortly thereafter. She remained on diuretics for several years. Occasionally she would have a flare-up, the lumbar puncture would be repeated, and again she would feel immediate relief as the extra fluid was taken off. Finally, with her weight at 150 pounds, she was taken off the diuretics and remained well.

CLUSTER HEADACHE

The cluster headache is a special type of headache. It is fairly rare in children, usually affecting people in their early twenties, but it has been described in patients as young as three years of age. Boys seem to be affected more than girls. Unlike migraine headaches, cluster headaches do not seem to run in families.

Cluster headaches, as the name implies, are headaches that seem to come in bouts. During a cluster, a child may experience several headaches a day, several days in a row. They may happen at the same time each day, and often occur at night. The headaches tend to be short, usually lasting several minutes to an hour but occasionally longer. They are sharp pains that usually are worst around the eye, affecting just one side of the head at a time and tending to stay on the same side. The affected eye itself may look red, teary, and irritated. There may be sweating and facial redness on the affected side.

These are very painful episodes, and, if affected, your child will usually be very uncomfortable. He will probably appear restless and agitated, and he may not want any help from you. Unlike migraine headaches, there is usually no associated light sensitivity or nausea, and your child will probably not want to sleep.

Example of a child with cluster headaches

Eighteen-year-old Michael had just entered his first year of college and was having a great time. However, he began to have terrible attacks of headaches. The first few days he would have a headache every night at eight o'clock, no matter what he was doing. They were short, only fifteen minutes long, but intensely painful. It would be as though somebody was driving a knife through his right eye, and his eye would water and become very red. The pain would come on quickly, without warning, and disappear quickly. During the time he had the pain, he would pace around outside in the cold night air. He would take some ibuprofen for the pain, but felt that the headache probably disappeared on its own; by the time he got to the medication, the headache would already be subsiding.

As the days went on, he began to have more headaches, several a day. They tended to happen at the same time every day. After two weeks, the headaches went away. Over the next few years, Michael had several clusters of headaches such as these. His doctor treated him with a preventative headache medication that helped somewhat, and an injectable medication that helped relieve the pain quickly once it started.

HEADACHES DUE TO GENERAL MEDICAL PROBLEMS

A variety of medical problems can cause headaches. Most parents are very familiar with headaches accompanying common upper respiratory illnesses, gastroenteritis, and "the flu."

There are some other conditions which tend to trigger headaches. Anemia, or a low red blood cell count, can be associated with headaches. Anemia is overall less common in children than adults, tends to give very dull headaches, and may be associated with a general feeling of exhaustion. Adolescent girls who have heavy and/or long periods are most at risk for anemia. A particular type of blood disease that causes anemia, sickle cell disease, may lead to bleeding in the brain, causing a severe and sudden headache.

Conditions that cause low levels of thyroid hormone (hypothyroidism) may also cause nonspecific headaches. Most children who have this problem also have other associated symptoms such as weight gain or a feeling of always being cold.

HEADACHES WITH PSYCHIATRIC PROBLEMS

Many physicians have identified an association between headaches and certain psychiatric disorders. Major depression is the most commonly identified disorder, but people with headaches also seem to have a higher proportion of panic disorders and anxiety disorders than would be expected by chance alone. Nobody is quite certain exactly where the cause lies.

Depression is fairly common in children, and is frequently seen in adolescents of both sexes. For your child, it may be unclear whether the depression is causing the headaches, or the headaches are causing the depression. Both situations may be occurring at once. Depression seems to be particularly common in headaches that have gone on a long time (days, weeks, or longer). The bottom line is that if your child is depressed and has headaches, both problems may need to be attended to. This can be done with counseling, biofeedback, and medications.

HEADACHES AND MEDICATIONS

Sometimes, the medications used to treat general medical and psychiatric problems can cause headaches as a side effect. Almost any medication can be the culprit. If your child's headaches started after he was given a new medication, check with your doctor about the possibility that this could be related. Don't discontinue the medication without first checking with the doctor who prescribed it.

COLLOID CYSTS

Headaches caused by colloid cysts are rare, but they can be quite dangerous. A cyst is a fluid-filled, noncancerous growth, and "colloid" refers to the type of fluid found in a particular type of cyst. Colloid cysts grow in the center of the brain's ventricular system and can block the flow of the fluid within the system. Colloid cysts are suspected when a child has headaches that change with head position, called positional headaches—especially if the headaches worsen with lying down. The cyst can be diagnosed by a CT scan, and the cyst must be surgically removed.

SLEEP APNEA

Sleep apnea—a condition where breathing is interrupted during sleep—usually occurs if a child has an obstruction to the flow of air from the mouth and nose to the lungs. This can be caused by big tonsils or adenoids or for other reasons. Usually, the child will be a "snorer," and you will hear the child stop breathing for periods of about fifteen to thirty seconds at a time while he sleeps. This can cause nonspecific daytime headaches and fatigue.

CHIARI I MALFORMATION

Chiari I malformation is a particular type of anatomical abnormality that has received mention in the popular media recently. In this condition, the back of the brain (the cerebellum) is positioned lower than normal, compressing the brainstem. This can happen with varying degrees of severity. See Figure 3 for an example of this condition.

For some children, this condition is thought to cause headaches. It is treated surgically, often by taking out a small piece of the skull in the back of the head to try to decompress the area.

Surgery for this condition solely for the purpose of treating headaches is controversial; however, if certain neurologic symptoms such as difficulty walking, numbness, or weakness are present, surgery would more likely be recommended. However, most children with Chiari I malformation have only a mild case

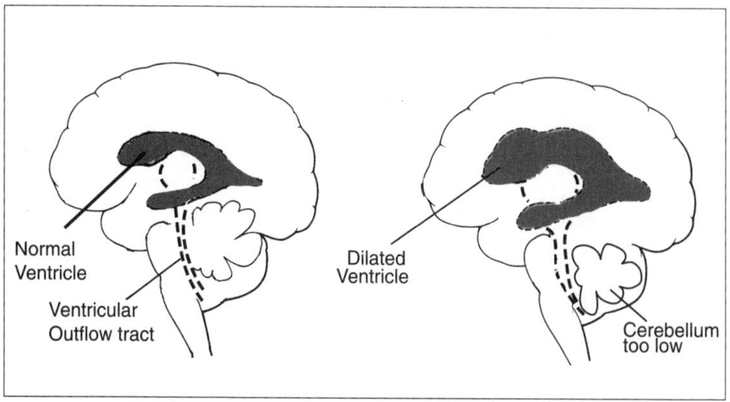

Figure 3. On the left, a normal brain. The ventricles are of normal size. On the right, a Chiari malformation is present with a low cerebellum compressing the ventricular outflow tract and causing dilatation of the ventricles.

and should not be operated upon. Many times, the Chiari I malformation will not be the cause of their headaches at all.

• • •

These are just some of the many causes of headache in children. It will often take a combination of parental observation, the child's ability to express his feelings, and patient work by medical personnel to help diagnose why a child has headaches.

CHAPTER 3

More Than Pain: Migraine

What is a migraine headache? What makes it different from other types of headaches? Despite the fact that migraine headaches were described in the medical literature as far back as 1200 B.C., these are still difficult questions to answer. They remain important, however, because migraines are a very common type of headache, even in children.

Due to many factors, estimates vary on how common migraine is. The most important problem is that it is hard to agree on just exactly what a migraine headache is, and what may distinguish it from other types of headaches, such as tension-type. Although for research purposes there are standard criteria for defining what is or is not a migraine headache, many physicians feel that those criteria are too narrow for use in a regular doctor's office. That is, many headaches that probably are migraines do not fit those criteria. To add to the difficulty, many people who have headaches may not seek help from a doctor—and certainly most do not see doctors who are keeping or reporting statistics. However, it is agreed that migraine is either the most common type of headache syndrome or the second most common (after tension-type), and it may be increasing in frequency.

In children, statistics are especially difficult to come by because very little information is available. It is estimated that between 7 and 18 percent of children experience migraines. We do know that boys tend to develop their migraines earlier than girls but then seem to outgrow them faster. That is, boys tend to develop their migraines in their prepubertal years (mostly from the ages of six to ten), girls around the time of puberty (eleven to fifteen years of age). However, in adults several studies have shown that only about 8 percent of men continue to have migraines, whereas about 18 percent of women will have them. For females, migraine tends to be a problem that sticks around a long time, whereas males have a better chance of outgrowing it.

My child is too young to have migraines!

This is one of the most common responses in parents when their children are diagnosed with migraines. Most people have a perception that migraines only happen to adults. However, more than half of adults who experience migraine had their first attack in childhood, and it is thought that even infants experience migraines. So, no one is "too young" to have migraines. In fact, about a third of children with migraines had their headaches start before they were five, and two-thirds by age seven. According to some studies, 10 percent of school-age children suffer from migraines, and up to 20 percent of teenage girls may be affected.

THE GENETICS OF MIGRAINES: WHY SHOULD YOUR CHILD DEVELOP THEM?

The genes your child inherited are thought to play a large part in whether your child develops migraine headaches. Migraines tend to run in families, and one study has estimated that approximately 90 percent of children diagnosed with them will have other family members who are also affected. You can help your doctor by coming to the appointment with some knowledge of your family's medical history. You may need to ask your relatives directly whether they are prone to migraines or headaches in general. Remember, many people may not even mention their headaches to their doctor, and the headaches generally do not require hospitalization and visits from relatives. Therefore, the knowledge of these headaches may not be passed on through the family. (In contrast, people are much more likely to know about their relatives' histories of cancer, diabetes, strokes, heart attacks, and other illnesses.)

Remember, though, that just because your child may be prone to migraines does not mean that his headaches are migraines. This should not be assumed just because of family history; rather, family history is only one piece of information that can be used as supporting evidence. Your child's headaches should be checked out by qualified medical personnel.

It's also important to remember that just because your child is prone to migraines does not mean that your child will actually have the headaches or that she has to suffer through them. Environmental and dietary manipulations and other preventative strategies, as well as a number of new and effective medications, may make your child's symptoms quite benign. If you are reading this book because your child suffers from migraines, there is a good chance that you have suffered from migraines as well—perhaps as a child, perhaps starting as an adult. If your headaches were severe as a child, that does not mean that your child's will have to be. This is an important point, because many people just assume that their child will have to go through the same difficulties they did. If this attitude is transmitted to your child, your child will approach his headaches with a lack of hope and a feeling of being out of control. Hopelessness and helplessness are two factors that may contribute to more intense headache experiences. (See Chapter 1 for a full discussion of how children perceive their pain.)

YOUR LITTLE MIGRAINE SUFFERER MAY GROW UP TO BE FAMOUS!

Examples of famous people who grew up with and suffered from migraines include:

Benjamin Franklin	Charles Darwin
Sigmund Freud	Julius Caesar
Abraham Lincoln	Thomas Jefferson
Frederic Chopin	Peter Tchaikovsky
Karl Marx	Virginia Woolf
Lewis Carroll	George Bernard Shaw
Edgar Allan Poe	Stephen King

Of these, Lewis Carroll may have made particular use of his migraine experiences in his famous book, *Alice in Wonderland.* Alice's experiences in feeling larger or smaller are probably based on a fairly unusual phenomena experienced by migraine patients called metamorphopsia, which involves changes in the perception or shape of objects.

THE SYMPTOMS OF MIGRAINES

Migraines have a variety of symptoms that your child could be experiencing. As discussed earlier in the chapter, it is difficult to say exactly what symptoms constitute a migraine, and many of the criteria were designed for headaches that occur in adults. However, although many people commonly use the term migraine just to mean "a very bad headache," there are some frequently found symptoms that can suggest that your child is suffering specifically from migraines. No one child is going to suffer from all of these features, but if some are prominent in your child's headache pattern then the diagnosis needs to be carefully considered.

Migraines are usually discussed in terms of four phases: the prodrome, the aura, the headache, and the resolution.

The first phase: the prodrome. The prodrome refers to a period of time before the headache itself begins. For some children headaches will come on so quickly that this phase is not even really experienced, but other children can have a prodrome that lasts for hours or even longer. In the prodrome period, children may act differently than their usual pattern of behavior. Older children may be able to describe what they are experiencing, but in younger children (especially those who are preverbal) a parent may see only nonspecific irritability or some vague abdominal complaints (a "tummy ache"). While over half of adults who suffer from migraines can identify some prodromal complaints, it is unclear what percentage of children may do so. Clearly, however, some children will have them.

Older children may have pronounced differences in mood. Usually they will appear more depressed or withdrawn, but occasionally will seem hyperexcitable or even euphoric. They may have trouble settling down to concentrate on their work and may give off a general sense of restlessness. Some children will seem drowsy or have seemingly uncontrolled, frequent yawning. Changes in eating patterns are frequently observed—eating a lot, losing a previously good appetite, or craving a particular food. Thirst can be prominent. Vomiting can occur, and bowel habits can change (to either constipation or diarrhea).

Until an association with headaches is made, these symptoms can really be puzzling to parents. Some of the problems seem to point to problems in other body systems, and care may be initially directed there. For example, if a child were to have prominent vomiting or bowel changes, he may have X rays and other studies made of his gastro-intestinal tract. It might be surmised that his headaches are a result of his stomach problems, rather than the other way around. A headache diary (see Chapter 5 and

Appendix A) or a family history of migraine may be helpful in identifying prodromal symptoms and establishing their relationship to the headache.

Example of a Migraine in a Four-Year-Old Child

Molly was generally a darling, cherubic little girl. She was her Daddy's pride and joy—most of the time. Once or twice a month she would go through some uncontrollable screaming fit of temper, throw up, and then seem to be fine. Nobody could understand what would trigger these events, and they would seem to come on quite suddenly. They often came on in department stores, and initially her parents were told that Molly just couldn't handle crowds very well. That didn't make much sense to Molly's parents, who noted that most of the time Molly seemed to handle strangers and other crowded areas with ease. Her parents did not know what to do when Molly would start one of these episodes. She was simply wild during these events, and would throw herself on the floor. When her dad would try to pick her up she would fight like crazy.

After the family had been through about ten of these episodes and had tried a variety of behavioral interventions ("let her cry," "give her lots of attention," "give her no attention,") a medical workup was started. An X ray of her stomach came back normal. During the appointment a family history of migraine on Molly's maternal side was identified, although Molly's mother's headaches were never anything like what Molly was displaying. Molly's mother remembered episodes of prominent head pain, beginning around age thirteen. They had actually improved after college, to the point where Molly's mother had almost forgotten about them. Molly was placed on a migraine preventive agent, which worked beautifully. Molly again became the apple of Dad's eye (even in stores—especially because Dad was able to blame the whole thing on Mom's genes!).

Molly was weaned off her medication after about nine months. Her parents continued to wonder why this would occur in department stores, but never really found out. What was the migraine trigger? The lighting? The odor in the perfume department? It always remained a mystery.

The second phase: the aura. The aura refers to neurological symptoms—visual complaints, sensory complaints, problems with weakness, even difficulty with talking—that can occur in migraines. This usually occurs just before the headache pain starts, but can occur during the headache. In addition, auras may occur *without* the headache.

Many adults who have experienced auras (or know someone who has) are under the mistaken impression that having an aura is a requirement for the diagnosis of migraine, that if the headache does not involve an aura it isn't a migraine. Auras are, in fact, fairly uncommon in children, happening approximately 5 percent of the time or less. In addition, many children will have the aura phase only rarely, having a "regular" headache most of the time.

Auras can be quite scary for children, their parents, and their physicians, especially the first time they are experienced. Put yourself in the position of this twelve-year-old girl experiencing her first aura:

> I was taking a math test that I had been studying very hard for. All of a sudden I began to see a black spot out of my right eye which grew until I could no longer see anything to my right. I didn't know what to do, it was the middle of the test, and I was scared I was going blind. I went out to get some water. When I came back the teacher said I looked pale and sent me to the nurse' s office. They called 911.

Most auras seem to be visual in nature. The reason for this is unclear; the part of the brain that processes vision may be particularly prone to migraine.

Visual auras can take many forms. A common form in children is the appearance of tiny flashes of light (a phenomenon called photopsia). Others may see zig-zag or arc-shaped lines of white or shimmering colors (these are called fortification spectra). There may be a greyish patch in part or all of a field of vision: imagine looking through a video-camera lens that has a patch of Vaseline on it. A child may describe this as "blurry vision." Some children (as in the example of Amy) will have partial blindness; there may be a black or gray spot cutting out a portion of the image seen by either or both eyes (these spots are called scotomas). It is rare, however, to have total blindness. The scotomas may be surrounded by light or color. All of these visual events may be stable in size, or the child may feel that the various spots and shapes are moving or growing.

The more unusual visual disturbances can be quite interesting and reminiscent of *Alice in Wonderland* or the funhouse mirrors at an amusement park. Children can see things and people around them as being large, small, or otherwise misshapen. They can feel as though part of their body is distorted, such as one hand or leg growing larger. They can have the perception that things are moving away from them or toward them, or rotating. They may feel like they are behind a zoom lens of a camera, sometimes feeling close up and sometimes far away. As in amusement park mirrors, parts of a person's body that the child sees may be perceived as suddenly ballooning out, or the child may have the feeling that they or others around them are floating. Mosaic vision is a very rare phenomenon, where the visual field seems to be broken down into small facets. None of these visual changes are really hallucinations (seeing things that aren't really there), rather they are distortions of what the child is actually looking at. Time can also be distorted; children can have the perception that events around them are moving slowly or quickly.

As one could imagine, the more complicated these disturbances are, the harder it is for a child to describe them. In addition, hard as it is to believe, a child may actually be in denial that there is a big black patch in his visual field. He may not mention it to his parents, who are often very surprised if this information comes out at the doctor's office for the first time!

Example of a child with an unusual aura

Mallory was an only child, an honor student in sixth grade with high verbal abilities. Just past her thirteenth birthday, she began to have brief episodes that she described as her "slow-motion" episodes. In the office, she described them quite vividly. She would be doing her normal activities, and then for a few minutes would get the strange sensation that people around her were walking slowly, talking slowly, and that everything around her was slowing down. She herself felt trapped during the episode, and there was an overall sense of confusion and fear during the times they were occurring. At first, the episodes occurred once every few months, but then they began happening more and more frequently. When she was first seen for these episodes, she did not have any symptoms of headache with them. There was, however, a family history of migraine.

Mallory had a series of tests, including an MRI and an EEG (electroencephalogram—a test for seizure activity in the brain waves), all of which came back normal. By the time the tests were complete, she had begun to have headaches following many of her "slow-motion" episodes, and at that point she was started on an antimigraine medication regimen. She did very well, and over time she required less and less medication.

Besides visual changes, another common aura includes a feeling of dizziness or light-headedness. This has been reported in between 20 and 50 percent of patients. It commonly lasts through much of the headache phase, and can be quite disabling. Children may feel like the room is spinning around them (a sensation known as vertigo), but more commonly have a general feeling of being "woozy," as though they had just stood up too quickly. These episodes of dizziness can occur without any headache and can last for days.

Strange sensations over the body can also be auras. Usually a sensory aura will consist of numbness or tingling in the hand or face. It may start on one or both sides of the body and may slowly migrate during the course of the aura. Painful sensations such as stomachaches (sometimes associated with vomiting) can also occur. As with the visual changes, children may not mention these symptoms unless specifically asked.

Motor changes are more easily observed in your child, and if severe they can be quite frightening. Statistically it is rare, but some children will have episodes of apparent paralysis on one side of the body, mimicking a stroke. Usually the first time this happens, the child is rushed to the emergency room for a CT scan, a quite appropriate response. However, if this happens several times and especially if it is followed by headache, it may eventually be recognized as part of a child's migraine symptoms. More commonly children will talk about feeling generally weak, often described by them as "my legs feel heavy."

Changes in thinking can occur. Children may have difficulty with speaking or other language disturbances, and they may have difficulty concentrating. They may appear confused and unable to recognize familiar people and situations around them. They may have a feeling of déjà vu. One of my patients had an aura of déjà vu followed by headache, and interestingly her mother had the same symptoms around her own migraines as well.

The older a child is, the better he will be able to describe these changes, but they can really present confusing symptoms to parents and doctors. Further testing such as an electroencephalogram (EEG) to rule out seizures, or an MRI test may be ordered. However, sometimes the diagnosis only becomes clear over time, as these episodes are repeated over and over and other migraine symptoms (such as the actual headache) begin to occur with them. A family history of migraines can also help to clarify that the symptoms your child is experiencing may indeed be migraine auras.

The third phase: the headache. Adult migraine headaches are classically one-sided (occurring on only one side of the head), throbbing, and severe. The pain experienced by children under twelve years old is not usually described like that, but older children have a higher tendency to have the more classic symptoms. Most young children, when asked where the pain is, will point to the middle of their forehead. "Behind my eyes" or "on top of my head" are other common responses. In older children and teenagers, migraine pain will typically shift from one side of the head to another. Alternatively, it may shift from the front of the head to the back (or vice-versa). This shifting can occur during a single headache or change from headache to headache. This sort of movement is generally reassuring and quite suggestive of migraine pain (as opposed to pain from other causes of headaches).

It may be difficult for your child to describe his headache more particularly than "it hurts." Children older than seven years of age may be able to distinguish "throbbing" or "pulsing" from "tight" or "stabbing," but it's sometimes difficult even for adults to give a precise description. Children may use concrete words such as "like a hammer" or "pounding," and may pantomime a hitting motion. However, since this can be so variable, it is often the least important characteristic to ask about. The child's pain may be worsened by exercise or other activities or even just moving his head. The build-up of pain can be very fast in some children and develop more slowly in others.

Migraine pain may not always be particularly severe. Often, children will talk about their "migraine headaches" and their "regular headaches." By this, they mean that some of their headaches are severely painful and the rest are less so. Both kinds will usually respond to the same antimigraine medications and interventions, and both may represent migraines. Remember, though, that different factors can affect the child's perception of pain, such as the responses of parents or others around them, activities they are doing or want to do, and previous experience (see Chapter 1 for a full discussion).

The length of time that the pain lasts can likewise be quite variable. Most of the time, migraines in children last an hour or more (migraines in adults tend to last longer). However, some children will describe pain lasting on the order of only a few minutes. Although these brief headaches are so short and quick, they probably do represent a variant of migraines. Some children who start with brief headaches will find that their headaches become longer.

Parents may not only see that their child appears to be in pain, but that other features begin to manifest themselves during this phase. Children are often described as becoming pale during a headache, with dark circles under their eyes; children may also appear flushed. Often times, children will feel like throwing up or actually do so (sometimes repetitively). Throwing up may make the child feel better. Some children will have tender areas on their scalp, and they notice that pressing these areas can make the headache worse. Children may avoid bright lights if the lights make their headache worse (called photophobia). They may additionally or alternatively avoid loud sounds (phonophobia) or may be sensitive to smells. The child may seek out or be most comfortable in a dark, quiet room. Children frequently will want to lie down or sleep during the headache phase, and sleeping will often make the headache go away. It can be very alarming to a parent to hear their child, who normally vigorously resists going to bed, ask to go to sleep. Children are often cranky and irritable during the headache itself.

Also during the headache, as during the aura phase, some children will have the unusual symptom of not being able to move one side of their body (called hemiplegia) or have numbness in part of the body. These symptoms, although rare, can be quite frightening to the child and the people around him; it may look as though he is having a stroke.

Most of the time, migraine headaches will occur during the day when the child is awake. They can occur in the morning or afternoon, but most commonly appear toward the end of the day. It is less common for the headache to actually wake a child from sleep, and if this is happening it may push your child's doctor to do further studies. Many times, children will have their headache toward the end of the school day. This can be caused by a number of factors. Some children's migraines may be triggered by hunger or thirst, and this would be the time of day when this is most likely to occur (especially if the child has skipped lunch). Scheduling a snack may help a child avoid such headaches. General stress from school or stress from certain classes could also trigger the headaches. Headaches are also sometimes worsened as the children are coming home on the bus, because children with migraine also tend to have a tendency toward motion sickness.

The fourth phase: the resolution. For some children, when the headache pain starts to get better it happens almost instantaneously and completely. Their headache leaves, and everything is back to normal. For other children, resolution may occur over hours. During this period they may feel slightly better, but often they feel that if they overdo it, the headache will come back. One of my patients has described this stage as "bits of the headache try to come back, then go away again."

Many children will feel quite tired after a migraine attack, and often sleep has contributed to the headache going away. It may be difficult for them to concentrate. They may feel depressed and irritable, but others will actually feel euphoric.

MIGRAINE VARIANTS

Some children experience symptoms that are thought to be related to migraines, but they do not experience the headaches (or they experience the headache later in life). For example, some experience repeated bouts of dizziness. Others experience visual symptoms (described above in the section on migraine auras) that do not progress to the headache phase.

Another variant, thought to only happen in children, is called *acute confusional migraine.* Children who suffer from this type of migraine experience episodes of confusion, where they don't seem to know what's going on around them. For example, one three-year-old boy who experienced an acute confusional migraine was fine when his parents dropped him off at day care. However, the day care called the parents mid-morning to report that their child was acting quite strangely. Indeed, when his parents picked him up, he did not seem to know who they were. When he got home, he did not appear to know where he was. This episode lasted about two hours, and then the child was back to normal. He had several more spells over the next two years.

A child with recurrent episodes of confusion needs a physician to evaluate him, in all likelihood with an electroencephalogram (EEG). EEGs are tests that are used to detect seizure activity in the brain. Seizures can sometimes look like episodes of confusion.

A frequently discussed migraine variant is called an *abdominal migraine.* Children who suffer from this have repeated bouts of abdominal pain or vomiting for which no medical or psychological cause can be identified. Even though the child may not suffer headache pain, there is thought to be a possible link between these symptoms and migraine. There are good reasons for this: recurrent abdominal pain or recurrent vomiting runs in families just as migraines do, and in such cases a family history of migraine can often also be identified.

A child with recurrent abdominal symptoms first needs a thorough investigation of his gastrointestinal tract. If this does not show a cause for any of the symptoms, migraine could be a consideration. A CT scan of the head may be ordered, as tumors and other brain masses can lead to recurrent vomiting. Furthermore, as stress so commonly affects children by causing stomach pain, a psychological evaluation (and possible treatment) may also be helpful.

INTRACTABLE MIGRAINES

These are discussed at length in Chapter 7, but some children do develop migraines that last for many days, weeks, or longer. These are called by many names, including intractable migraines, migraine status, or status migrainosus. Such migraines can be difficult to manage, and they often require a variety of different approaches.

MIGRAINE TRIGGERS: WHAT WILL SET OFF A HEADACHE IN YOUR CHILD?

If your child is suspected of having migraines, it is important to look for triggers. (The topic of triggers is discussed more in Chapter 5.) In quite a few children, foods, stressors, or other aspects of the child's environment may trigger migraines. These triggers will be different for different children. For example, one father of a patient of mine noticed that the more sugar his child ate, the more migraines he had. After cutting out sugary cereals from the child's diet, the number of headaches the child complained of was greatly reduced. However, other children might respond to other types of changes in diet (or there may be no dietary triggers ever identified). Other commonly seen triggers include motion (riding in a car) or mild head injuries.

Migraines and head trauma

Children with migraine headaches should in general try to exercise and participate in sports activities as normally as possible. However, parents should be aware that the normal "head bumps" that occur during such activities can trigger migraines. Here is an example:

Jamie, fourteen years old, had had migraines for about a year, fairly well controlled on very low-dose preventative medication. However, during a basketball game at school, the back of her head neatly blocked a fast and forceful pass. She did not get knocked out, and she actually continued the game. However, as she was showering and getting dressed afterward, she had the sensation that she was seeing green spots. As she described it, "it was like I had stared at a light bulb too long and then looked away, and the spots followed everything." She developed headaches with nausea after about an hour. The next morning she felt normal, but by the afternoon she had the same sensations (except now with purple spots instead of green) lasting about two hours. She gradually got better over the next few days.

BIOLOGY OF A MIGRAINE HEADACHE

As stated earlier, we don't know exactly what goes on in and around the brain during a migraine attack (or, for that matter, during most headaches in general). Studying how a living brain works (or in this case, malfunctions) is not easy to do. It is only recently that we have been able to get real-time images of brains as they are functioning. Using new imaging techniques such as functional magnetic resonance imaging (fMRI), single photon emission CT (SPECT), and positron emission tomography (PET) scanning, we can now begin to understand which areas of the brain increase their blood flow or change their metabolism during an actual headache.

These techniques let us look at changes in relatively large areas of the brain. That is, at best they will look at changes in cubic centimeters of brain tissue (which contain millions of brain cells). They cannot determine much about what is going on at the level of the individual brain cell. However, advances in imaging techniques are coinciding with progress in genetics and new methods of drug development, both of which add their own unique contributions to understanding how headaches may start and propagate.

We understand more about the basic biology of migraine headaches than of other headache types, and it is described in the following paragraphs. Remember, though, that many headache types probably share common pathways.

The study of the biology of migraines has been conducted in adults. As there are probably some differences in general brain physiology between adults and children (not much is clear in this area), there are probably some differences in the biology of migraine in particular. The following information is the best available, and much of it is probably applicable to children, too.

• • •

The vascular theory. Until the last decade or two, the vascular theory of migraines was quite popular. The vascular theory of migraines blamed excessive dilatation of brain blood vessels, putting pressure on little nerves outside of the blood vessels and generating pain. The major medications for treating migraines, ergotamines, worked by constricting the blood vessels. However, nobody could explain why the blood vessels were dilating in the first place.

We now think that the cause of migraines is not the blood vessels themselves, but rather some other part of the brain. This part of the brain starts functioning differently, and it is this primary brain dysfunction that triggers changes in the blood vessels. Instead of the blood vessels being the primary culprits, the brain itself is the trigger. The sensation of pain is still thought to be generated by the blood vessels, but the underlying cause of the migraine is much more complex.

What are the actual chemical changes in the brain that start and propagate a migraine attack? Where in the brain are the changes occurring? This is just being figured out. Here are some theories.

The calcium hypothesis. It has long been recognized that migraine headaches tend to run in families. In the early 1990s, a gene for a particular migraine syndrome was actually discovered. The type of migraine disorder, familial hemiplegic migraine, is extremely rare, but the discovery of its genetic basis was quite important. Not only did it provide the first hard evidence that migraines could actually be coded into our genes, but finding the gene and learning more about exactly what it did enabled scientists to begin to figure out what cellular processes were involved in at least that particular type of migraine.

They found that the gene is involved in the process of how calcium is conducted into brain cells. Calcium is an ion that is required for normal cellular processing. The amount of calcium going into and out of a nerve cell is very tightly regulated. Therefore, the discovery brought up the possibility that migraines might be caused by problems in the gates that let calcium into the cells.

The theory is that most of the time the gates function normally, and during this time the headache sufferer is pain-free. However, certain triggers (diet or hormonal changes, for example) could "overload" or change the basic biology of these gates. In the people prone to headaches, the gates are more likely to dysfunction during those times, and headaches will start. (There is no correlation, however, between calcium in the diet and the calcium at these gates, and no one should try to alter their diet with the goal of trying to alter what is happening at these calcium gates.)

This is a relatively new theory about why some people are prone to migraines and others are not, and it explains how at least some of the people may inherit this tendency from their parents. It is, however, only a beginning. For one thing, nobody really knows how many migraine types (or other types of headaches) may work this way.

The serotonin factor. Besides calcium, there are many different chemicals involved in a migraine attack. One of the most important is a neurotransmitter called serotonin. Neurotransmitters are specialized molecules that transmit messages between nerve cells.

There have been several clues that serotonin is involved in migraine attacks. Some of the most important have come from patients' reactions to different types of medications that alter the levels of serotonin in the brain. Some medications that deplete serotonin are known to bring on migraine attacks, and others that increase serotonin are known to cure migraine attacks. Interestingly, sleep is a time when the brain systems that use serotonin are very active, which may be why when both adults and children (but particularly children) have a migraine, they will often fall asleep. When they wake up, the headache is often gone. It is possible that naturally elevated serotonin levels during sleep help the brain heal itself.

The most effective medications for migraine available today affect the serotonin system. These are discussed further in Chapter 4.

THE CYCLE OF A MIGRAINE

The prodrome: Where in the brain does a headache start? Before a migraine attack really starts, many people know it is going to happen. They might have changes in emotion—feelings of depression, irritability, or, in some cases, euphoria. They might feel particularly hungry or thirsty, or even a little more sleepy than usual. Because of this, researchers in migraine are particularly interested in the areas of the brain (such as the limbic system; see Figure 4) that control emotions, appetite, and sleepiness—could migraines start in these areas?

Another interesting feature that may give us a clue about where in the brain migraines start is the observation that some people have periodicity to their migraine attacks. That is, some people get the migraine attacks at very predictable, set intervals. For many women, migraines come predictably at the time of their menstrual cycle. For other people, they may come once in a set amount of calendar days—once every 137 days, for example. There are particular areas of the brain (such as one area called the

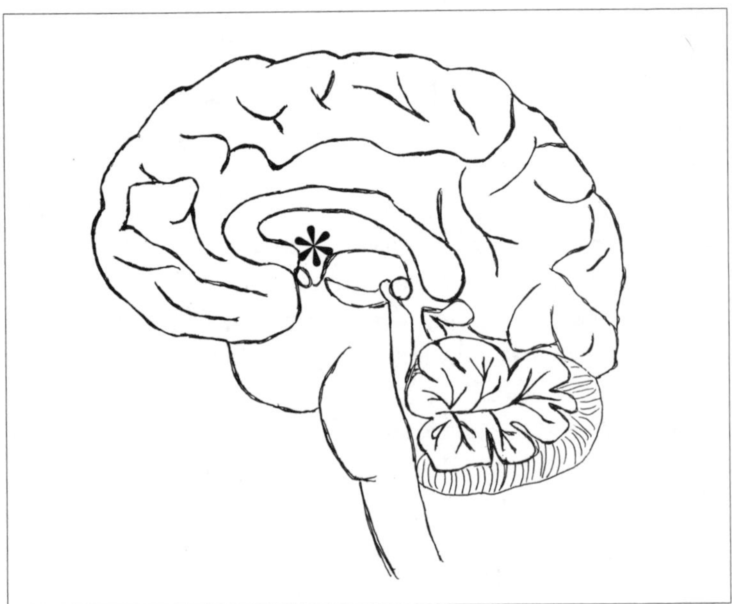

Figure 4. The asterisk marks the area where migraines may start, deep within the brain.

suprachiasmatic nucleus) that seem to keep track of time. Could those areas be involved with starting migraines?

Very little is actually understood about where the headaches may start, and the location may vary in different people. It is hoped that, the advances in imaging techniques described earlier will help to shed some light on this aspect. One of the biggest obstacles to studying this is having the person in the scanner at the time the headache starts!

The aura: How does the migraine move from where it started to a different part of the brain to cause these new symptoms? Most people who are thought to have migraines never actually experience one of the most characteristic features of them: the aura. As described above, there are many different types of auras: visual auras (such as seeing spots or flashing lights, or having blurry vision), sensory auras (such as numbness of an arm), or motor auras (such as weakness of an arm or leg).

The question here is, what is happening in the brain during the aura? It may be that different parts of the brain are more sensitive in certain people, so that after a migraine is initially triggered, changes in the brain occur that cause these auras. For example, it may be that in people with visual auras, the occipital lobes of the brain (where vision is normally processed) are hypersensitive. In these areas there appears to be a spreading decrease in electrical activity, which leads to a secondary decrease in blood flow to these areas (see Figure 5).

The headache: What causes the actual pain? So far, we have focused on what starts the headache and where it spreads. What, though, is causing the actual pain?

We know that the brain cells themselves do not generate pain. Some people even undergo brain surgery without anesthesia because the surgeon can actually cut out what he has to without any pain to the patient. Patients will be under anesthesia

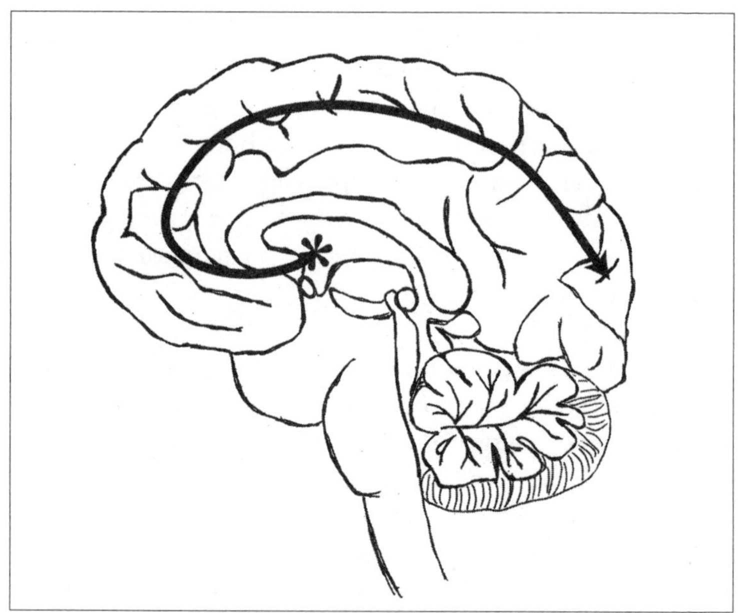

Figure 5: Starting deep within the brain, the biochemical changes involved in migraine then travel to the back of the brain (the occipital lobes).

while the surgeon is *getting to* the brain (making the incision in the scalp, skull, etc.), but cutting the brain itself does not hurt.

If headache is not "brain pain" then, where is the "ache" generated? Now we get back to the blood vessels. Surrounding many of the blood vessels that feed the brain is a network of nerve fibers. These nerve fibers all eventually come together in a cluster near the brainstem (a very deep area of the brain that, among other things, controls basic body functions such as heart rate and breathing) called the trigeminal ganglion. We know that, in contrast to the brain itself, these types of nerve fibers are very capable of generating pain. It is this network that is thought to be most responsible for the actual headache pain.

During the headache itself, blood flow to the brain is increased, and the diameter of the blood vessels gets bigger. These changes in the blood vessels affect the nerve fibers that surround them, and this probably triggers pain-generating substances to be released from these nerve cells. These pain-generating substances are then processed and interpreted by different areas in the brain, giving us the sensation that we know as "pain."

The end of the migraine: How does a headache end? The headache will either end by itself or with medication. Medications work on different parts of this system (see Chapter 4). An interesting question is how a headache, once started, will stop on its own. Nobody knows for sure, but the brainstem again appears to be involved, along with areas of the brain that are involved with generation of sleep.

Do headaches generate headaches?

Another way to phrase this question is: Are there any special changes in people who have a lot of headaches, as compared to those who have headaches once in a while? The answer has implications for how you might manage your child's headaches. What if the more headaches you have, the more headaches you are likely to have in the future? Your strategy would then shift toward preventing headaches from happening in the first place, not just dealing with them once they occur. Is there any evidence to support this?

Nearly all people who develop daily headaches have had a prior history of intermittent headaches. There is some evidence that this occurs because of neurochemical changes triggered by frequent headaches. Therefore, nobody can say how many headaches it might take to trigger other headaches in your child, but prevention of headaches could be very important for him, both now and in the future. Different strategies for preventing headaches, such as dietary changes, stress management, and medication, are described in the next two chapters.

To summarize, migraines may be the most frequent type of headache seen in children, even very young children. The symptoms of migraines are usually different from migraines typically seen in adults. Children's headaches are relatively shorter in length, are most likely to be centered in the forehead, and are frequently associated with nausea, vomiting, and a need to go to sleep. Children may have auras with their headaches, or the symptoms of the aura can occur without a headache. Migraines may be triggered by certain foods, stress, or environmental factors.

If you suspect your child has migraines, take heart! There are a number of very effective treatments, described in Chapters 4 and 5. Your child has an excellent chance of getting rid of those headaches.

CHAPTER
4

Take Two Aspirins... and Cross Your Fingers
Headache Medications

"She's banging her head against the wall, it hurts so bad. What can I give her to make her feel better?"

—Tired and worried mom of seven-year-old Amanda. Amanda had been suffering from a headache for three days straight.

If your child is having recurrent headaches, he or she will likely need medication for them at some point. But how does a parent know what to give? The number of medications for headache, both over-the-counter and prescription, is bewildering. There are literally hundreds of medications now available. It is difficult for anyone, including those in the medical field, to keep up with all of them.

This chapter will focus on some of the major medications used to treat headache. Your child's doctor may have other medications she favors.

Medications for headaches are used in a variety of ways. Some medications are used to prevent headaches from occurring in the first place. These medications will generally be given to people whose headaches happen frequently, or whose headaches tend to be quite severe. Preventative medications will be discussed in the first section of this chapter.

Other medications are used to stop a headache once it starts; these medications are called abortive mediations. This is the most common way people use medications for headaches. The abortive medications are discussed in the second section of the chapter.

The final section deals with potential drug interactions. It will answer questions of how and whether the different types of headache medications can be combined, and whether the medications could interact with other medications your child may be taking for other problems.

Many of the medications discussed here are not FDA-approved specifically for children's migraines, but they are widely used for children nonetheless. In many cases, studies done outside the FDA have proved their safety and efficacy. If you have concerns about this point, please be sure to discuss them with your child's physician.

The medications discussed in this chapter are useful for a variety of headache types, but they are most commonly used for migraine headaches and tension-type headaches. Some are prescription medications; some are over-the-counter medications. You and your doctor may use just one medication or a combination of several to come up with an optimal treatment strategy for your child.

PREVENTATIVE MEDICATIONS

Often the best way to deal with headaches is to prevent them from happening in the first place. This may be accomplished by avoiding dietary or other environmental triggers (see Chapter 5), but often parents will not be able to identify particular triggers for their child's headache. In these cases, preventative medications become very important.

Your child's doctor may bring up the idea of taking a daily preventative medication if your child's headaches are "frequent enough." How frequent is that? The question becomes, at what point are the benefits of taking a daily medication worth the potential side effects of doing so? The medication would have to be taken every day, whether your child is having headaches or not, for a certain period of time, until the child is headache-free (or close to it). The idea is to break the cycle of the headaches. After the headaches have been under control for a period of time (typically for a few months), the child would be slowly weaned off the medicine, in the hope that he would remain headache-free.

Generally, if your child is having several headaches per month, this strategy should at least be considered. If the headaches are brief or respond easily to simple over-the-counter medications, you may not feel that a daily medication is "worth it," unless your child is having headaches even more frequently (for example, several headaches per week). However, if your child's headaches tend to be severe (knocking him out for days at a time) and they are unresponsive to treatment, even infrequent headaches may be enough to start him on a preventative medication, at least until more effective strategies are found.

If your child is having headaches every day, these medications may be employed to break this daily cycle. You and your child's doctor will then have to come up with a plan of how long to keep him on the medication after the daily headache improves.

Specific medications will be described below, but here are some guidelines regarding overall use of these agents.

1. *First, try to start at the lowest possible dose.* This will need to be discussed with your child's doctor. When you are making your child take a medication every day, even when he is feeling well, the last thing you want is to introduce new side effects from the medication. Many side effects can be avoided if the medication is given in low doses and increased slowly. If side effects occur, going back and increasing the dosage even more slowly is often a good strategy. Some people are just more sensitive to side effects than others, and there is usually no way to predict this in advance. With children of all ages, it is best to avoid side effects in the first place if possible. Once a child gets it in his head that the medication makes him feel sick, it can be difficult to get him to take it.

2. *Second, have patience.* It is important for patients, families, and doctors to all remember that these medications may take several weeks to a couple of months to work to their fullest potential. If you want your child to be on the lowest possible medication dose, then you need to wait for the medication to have a chance to take effect. Otherwise, you and your doctor will probably start to give your child more and more medication, thinking that the lower doses do not work. You may even give up on the medication altogether. Depending, of course, on how severe your child's headaches are, you may not be able to wait a long time for the medication to work, and you may need to increase the dose relatively quickly. This needs to be discussed with your doctor. However, if you can wait and go slowly, it is probably in your child's best interest to do so. Be sure to ask your child's doctor how long he expects it will be before you can judge whether the medication is working.

3. *Finally, if these medications are to be effective,* they have to be taken consistently. Some medications will need to be taken once a day, and others more frequently. Be honest with your doctor. If there is no way you can envision your child taking a three-times-a-day medication for whatever reason—your schedule, your child's schedule, your child's strong aversion to taking medication—ask your doctor if there's an alternative medication that may have an easier dosing schedule. Don't have your child take the medication less frequently than prescribed, or "bunch up" the medication doses into one mega-dose that you give once a day. If your child is going to go through the trouble of being on a daily medication, at least the medication should be given the optimal chance of working with a minimum of side effects. Taking less than prescribed will make the medication less likely to work, and "bunching up" the doses will likely lead to side effects.

When you and your doctor do come up with a schedule that should work for you and your child, do your very best to try to stick to it. Give the medication at the same time each day, and tie it in to something that your child never misses, something that you can use as a "cue" to remind you about the medication. For example, if your child always brushes his teeth in the morning, give the medication to your child at that time, with the bottle clearly visible near the toothbrush so you don't forget. In contrast, if your child only sporadically eats breakfast, keeping the medication near the breakfast table would likely lead to missed doses.

Optimal strategies for giving a child preventative medication for headaches

The following points are discussed more fully in the text above, but this summary will hopefully be a handy jumping-off point for discussions with your child's doctor about the medications he is prescribing:

- *Start low.* Ask your child's doctor if this is the lowest possible dose to start your child on. If not, why not?
- *Go slow.* Remember that these medications generally will not cure your child's headache disorder quickly—they may take a few weeks to work. Try to be patient. Increase the dosage as slowly as possible, working with your child's doctor.
- *Take the medications as directed.* With the help of your child's doctor, come up with a medication schedule that will work with your family's schedule. Then, try to stick with it as conscientiously as possibly. If you accidentally miss a dose, use this as an opportunity to review what cues you and your child use to remember to take the medication.

Here are some of the more common types of preventative medications. Mechanisms of action (when known) will be discussed, as well as some of the more commonly seen side effects. This is by no means a comprehensive list of all the potential side effects of every medication. Also note that in the following sections, you will see drugs listed by two names. The first name is the name of the generic medication, the second (in parenthesis) is the trade name.

Beta-blockers. This is a very widely used class of medications, usually a good first choice for migraine prevention. These medications are generally very effective in migraine prevention—up to 80 percent of people who take them see their migraine frequency reduced by at least half. In addition, some of them have a very convenient dosing schedule: once a day. They have been used to prevent migraines for many years, although originally they were developed as a medication to lower high blood pressure. They should not, though, have any effect on your child's blood pressure unless the dose gets too high.

The major side effects of the beta-blockers are sleepiness and/or dizziness. Some children may also have problems exercising vigorously on this medication, as it tends to keep the heart rate on the lower side. Occasionally mood changes (such as depression) are seen. However, most children are able to take this kind of medicine very well, with minimal to no side effects. Starting low and increasing the dose slowly will help avoid side effects.

Doctors think that this medication works to prevent migraines in a number of ways. It has potential effects on stabilizing blood vessel walls, and may also affect neuro- transmitters in the brain such as serotonin, which is implicated in migraines.

These medications should not be given to children who have asthma, diabetes, congestive heart failure, or Raynaud's syndrome. If your child has any of these conditions, remind your doctor about them.

The most commonly prescribed beta-blockers have the following names: propranolol (Inderal), nadolol (Corgard), atenolol (Tenormin), and metoprolol (Lopressor).

Seizure drugs. Several of the medications that are useful in stopping seizures also have turned out to be effective in stopping migraines. Nobody knows exactly why that is, but it has been known for years that people who have seizures are more likely to have migraines, and vice-versa. Probably the medications are acting on some common chemical pathways involved in both problems.

There are different kinds of seizure drugs, and quite a few of them are thought to be useful in treating migraines. Phenytoin (Dilantin) and carbamazepine (Tegretol, Carbatrol) are among the oldest, but they may be a little less likely to work than some of the newer medications. Of the newer medications, valproic acid (Depakote) and gabapentin (Neurontin) seem to be fairly effective. Between the two, valproic acid is probably more likely to be effective, but it is also more likely to have side effects.

Valproic acid's most common side effects are stomachaches, sleepiness, and dizziness, all of which are usually worse at the beginning of therapy and will wear off if treatment is continued. It can also cause weight gain, tremors, and hair loss. It can have detrimental effects on the female reproductive system; it may cause or exacerbate a condition called polycystic ovaries, and should not be used if there is a potential for pregnancy. In some rare cases, it has been known to affect a person's blood count (especially platelets, which help the blood clot) and liver, so blood tests to monitor these aspects need to be done on a routine basis. This can be a scary medication to start for these reasons, but having stated all these potential problems, valproic acid is thought to be a safe medication for the vast majority of people who take it. The medication has been prescribed on a twice- or thrice-daily dosing schedule, but a new extended-release form was recently issued for once-a-day dosing.

Gabapentin's side effects are mainly sleepiness and dizziness, and sometimes include some stomach upset that usually improves over time. Gabapentin has an added benefit of not interacting with any other medications. However, it really should be taken three times a day, which is hard for many patients. As of this writing, two of the newest seizure drugs are being tried more frequently for headache prevention. Topamax (Topiramate) is showing promise in small studies of adult headache patients. Unlike many medications, topamax tends to make patients lose weight (seen as a benefit by some). Keppra (Levetiracetam), released at the end of 2000, is also showing some potential benefits. Overall, Keppra seems to be a fairly well-tolerated medication.

Calcium-channel blockers. Calcium-channel blocker medications, like beta-blockers, are a kind of blood pressure medication that has been useful in the prevention of migraines and cluster headaches. Like the beta-blockers, these medications also work in a variety of ways. They probably affect the release of serotonin and other neurotransmitters, and in addition they may change the calcium concentration in and around the brain cells, which likely would have a number of effects. The medications probably also cause stabilization of the size of blood vessels. Calcium-channel blocking medications should not cause changes in your child's blood pressure, though, unless the dose is too high.

The most common side effects of this medication are constipation, fatigue, and dizziness. In some people, this medication can worsen headaches. On the plus side, many of these medications can be given just once a day.

Names of commonly used calcium-channel blockers include verapamil (Calan, Isoptin), nifedipine (Procardia), and diltiazem (Cardizem).

Antidepressants. Several different classes of antidepressant medication have been used to prevent migraines. The neurochemical changes generated by these medications treat the migraine disorder itself; a person does not have to be depressed for these medications to work against their migraines. Giving these medications to children who are not depressed usually does not alter their mood; however, if a child has both depression and migraines, the medication could be beneficial on both fronts.

There are two major classes of antidepressant medications in use for migraine prevention. The medications that have been around the longest are the tricyclic antidepressants. The tricyclic antidepressants probably work by affecting a variety of neurotransmitters. They have the benefit of usually being given just once a day, but can have a variety of side effects including sleepiness, dry mouth, constipation, and weight gain. Particularly at higher doses, they have the potential of inducing abnormalities of heart rhythm; your child's doctor may order an electrocardiogram (EKG) prior to starting him on the medication to make sure there are no baseline problems. They do have a number of drug interactions, so if your child is on other medications, be sure to remind the doctor. Tricyclic antidepressants overall are inexpensive medications, and can be quite helpful in some children if the side effects are tolerable. The most commonly used tricyclic antidepressants are nortriptyline (Pamelor), amitriptyline (Elavil), imipramine (Tofranil), and doxepin (Sinequan).

The second and newer class of antidepressants is the selective serotonin reuptake inhibitors (SSRIs). Although the name implies a particular mechanism of action, these drugs in reality do not just work by altering the serotonin systems of the brain; they, too, have effects on other neurochemicals. They tend to have fewer side effects than the tricyclic antidepressants, but they may not be as effective for migraine prevention. Side effects of the SSRIs can include both sleepiness and hyperactivity, dry mouth, increased anxiety, and decreased sexual drive (the latter is not usually an issue for children, and is seen as a benefit by some parents of teenagers!). They do not affect the heart rhythm, as sometimes seen with the tricyclic antidepressants. The medication is generally given once or twice a day, and some are available in liquid preparations that are useful for children who don't take pills well. One (Prozac) is now available in a very long-acting form that can be taken once a week. Besides paroxetine (Paxil), other names of SSRIs include fluoxetine (Prozac), sertraline (Zoloft), fluvoxamine (Luvox) and citalopram (Celexa). Venlafaxine (Effexor) is an SSRI-like medication that may actually be a little more effective than the SSRIs. It works on slightly different receptors, but the side effects are similar. New SSRIs and SSRI-like medications are becoming available at a rapid rate.

Antihistamines. Cyproheptadine (Periactin) is a common example of an antihistamine that, when prescribed on a daily basis, can help to prevent migraines. The drug probably works by blocking some of the actions of serotonin in the brain. Periactin is frequently prescribed for children, as it is felt to be a very safe medication. Side effects most commonly are sleepiness and dry mouth.

Riboflavin. Riboflavin, also known as vitamin B2, has been recently tested for migraine prevention in adults. Adults who take 400 mg of riboflavin daily over a four-month period had a 50 percent reduction in their headache frequency. Riboflavin is tempting to prescribe for children, because the side effects in adults are minimal—just a small amount of diarrhea and increased urination in a few patients. However, appropriate doses have not been identified for younger children, and efficacy has not been established. Riboflavin also is most commonly available only in 50 mg pills, and asking even a teenager to take eight pills a day to prevent migraines is usually asking too much.

Tips on taking daily medicines

It is hard enough for an adult to stick to a routine of taking a daily medication, especially when he is feeling well. It is even harder to take the medication two or even three times a day. So how do you get your child to do it?

Younger children will have to be supervised when taking the medication. Older children (twelve and up) can gradually be given the responsibility for taking the medication on their own, but parents of teenagers do need to be sure that their child is actually swallowing the medication. Therefore, it is best to link the medication to a time when the parent and child are spending time together.

When you are giving your child daily pills, it is sometimes hard to remember if they have taken the medication. The child, especially if she is young, may not be able to help you remember. If you can't remember whether you've given the medicine or not, you can get in a bind: should you skip the dose and risk a headache, or give a dose and risk side effects? Another problem with taking pills out of a bottle is that if there are two parents around, each may give the child a dose without the other being aware. Again, the child may not be much help in this situation.

It is best to get a daily pill box, which is usually an inexpensive plastic box with a compartment for every day of the week. This is available in nearly every pharmacy. Fill up the compartments once a week. It will then be clear if the dose was given or not. If there are two parents involved, it may be best to designate one parent as the medication-giver and the other as the "reminder" person. This may help avoid double dosing.

What if the child does not want to take the medication? Try your best to find out why. If the child talks about side effects, you may want to discuss this with his doctor to see if a dose alteration would be possible. If the child gives a variation on "I just don't want to!" remind him about how the headaches have been such a problem and kept him from so many wonderful activities. Talk about all the fun activities he can do when the medication is working. You may want to "bribe" the child with coins every time he takes the medication, and every week go buy something with the money. Giving the child a small amount of their favorite food or drink to take with the medications can also be effective. If your child is really giving you a hard time, talk with his doctor to make sure that there is no alternative medication that could be given fewer times a day.

ABORTIVE MEDICATIONS

What can your child take to stop a headache once one has begun? In contrast to the preventative medications discussed in the section above, the following medications are taken only at the onset of headache, rather than every day. As a matter of fact, nearly all of these medications, if taken daily, may lead to rebound headaches (see the section on rebound headaches in Chapter 2).

The goal of the medication is to stop the headache, preferably with minimal side effects. Hopefully, you and your child will be able to find a medication that works well for him, at least most of the time. Sometimes, a medication that has worked in the past may seem to stop working. In that case, you and your child's doctor will probably need to find some alternate treatments.

As a general rule, these medications are most effective if taken as close to the onset of a headache as possible. If the headache is allowed to flourish, it will be harder to get any of these medications to work. If your child is old enough to talk, explain to him that it is important for him to tell you (or another adult) if a headache is starting. Tell him not to wait until the headache is really bad. If your child is pre-verbal, try to be alert to what he usually looks like at the first onset of headache symptoms, and get the medication into him then.

The following are some specific examples of medications for quick relief of headache pain.

Over-the-counter medications. One of the major benefits of this class of medication is its widespread use. As these drugs are inexpensive and available without a prescription, they have been used by millions of children and are generally thought to be quite safe. Many of them also come in liquid forms convenient for dosing small children. However, even over-the-counter medications can be dangerous if taken too often or in too high a dose. For example, too much acetaminophen can cause serious liver damage. Too much ibuprofen can cause serious kidney damage. Follow the labels carefully, and be sure to let your child's doctor know that he is taking the medication. Many parents don't seem to regard these as "medicines" since they do not require prescriptions. However, they are actually quite potent. Over-the-counter medications include acetaminophen (Tylenol), ibuprofen (Advil, Motrin), naproxen (Naprosyn, Anaprox), acetaminophen/aspirin/caffeine combination pills (Excedrin Migraine), aspirin.

Acetaminophen (Tylenol) seems to affect how the brain perceives pain. It dulls the sensation of pain, but it does not have any effect on the basic underlying causes of the pain. Unlike ibuprofen or naproxen, which do treat inflammation, acetaminophen does not have anti-inflammatory effects. It may be taken as often as every four hours for a short period of time, but if taken for more than a few days in a row acetaminophen has the potential to cause rebound headaches.

Acetaminophen in combination with aspirin and caffeine forms a popular product called Excedrin Migraine. This can be very effective in treating migraines, but again must be used with caution. If used on a daily basis, Excedrin Migraine (and other similar caffeine-containing medications) can cause caffeine withdrawal headaches. These headaches are usually noticed in the morning, as the caffeine from the previous day "wears off" during the night, and the child wakes up with a headache. The child may then be given more Excedrin Migraine to treat the headache, continuing a vicious cycle.

Ibuprofen (Advil, Motrin) and naproxen (Naprosyn, Anaprox) are similar to acetaminophen, but are actually in a different class of medications. These medications are called nonsteroidal anti-inflammatory drugs (abbreviated NSAIDs). Unlike acetaminophen, they do have some anti-inflammatory properties. Like aspirin, however, they also work by dulling perceptions of pain. Some reports have suggested that, on the whole, they may be a little better than acetaminophen at treating migraines, but there were no major differences. If your child responds to acetaminophen well, there is no reason to try to switch. Ibuprofen and naproxen have the benefit of being a little longer-acting than acetaminophen; they are given every six to twelve hours instead of every four. They can also be given together with acetaminophen. Possible side effects of NSAIDs include stomach pain and nausea.

Aspirin is another medication available over the counter and proven effective in adults. Aspirin and products containing aspirin, however, are not usually given to children because some children have a very serious reaction when they are taking it—Reye's syndrome, which causes severe liver damage.

Tylenol with codeine and other narcotics. Narcotics can be quite effective in treating pain, but many problems are associated with them. They work by acting on special receptors in the brain to block the signals the brain uses to perceive pain. However, they can be quite addictive. For a child who may need pain relief off and on for years, this category of medications should be used as a last resort. Besides dependence on the medication, there are other possible side effects. Rebound headaches (see Chapter 2) can be a result of regular use of narcotic medications. They also tend to make children sleepy or "loopy," with the children acting dizzy or silly. Constipation and depression are other risks.

Examples of narcotic medications include codeine-containing medications, meperidine (Demerol), oxycodone-containing medications (various brand names including Percocet), hydrocodone-containing medications (various brand names including Vicodin), and butorphanol tartrate (Stadol; also available in a nasal spray).

Ergotamine medications. Extracts of ergot, a fungus that grows on rye plants, have been used to treat migraines for more than a hundred years. The most common extract used to treat migraines today is called ergotamine tartrate (Wigraine, Ergomar, and other brand names). Ergotamine medications probably work by a variety of methods, including blood vessel constriction, effects on serotonin, and anti-inflammatory actions.

Ergotamine medications are mostly used in teenagers and older children. They are not FDA approved for use in children, however. Some come in a rapidly disintegrating form (meaning that they quickly dissolve in the child's mouth) or a rectal suppository form (useful for treating a child who tends to throw up a lot as a result of his headaches). They should never be given to a teenage girl who might be pregnant.

Dihydroergotamine (DHE) is another type of ergotamine medication. It comes in a new form called Migranol, delivered as a nasal spray as well as an injectable solution. Experience shows that DHE may cause fewer side effects than ergotamine preparations. It can also be very useful in treating a headache that has been present for a long time (see the information on "Treatment of Intractable Headaches," page 115).

These medications, while they can be quite effective, do tend to have many side effects. The most common side effects are nausea and vomiting, but not infrequently people have reported chest pain and numbness and tingling in the arms and legs. Overuse can clearly cause rebound headaches.

Ergotamine medications should probably not be used for children who have numbness or weakness of their arms and legs during a migraine attack, or children who have very prolonged auras. There is a chance (although remote) that these kinds of medications could prolong such symptoms or even make them permanent, through their effects on constriction of the blood vessels.

Barbiturate-containing combination medications. There are a number of medications that have a weak barbiturate called butalbital in them. The butalbital is often combined with aspirin or acetaminophen and caffeine. These are marketed under a few different names, including Fiorinal, Esgic, and Phrenilin.

These medications can be helpful in stopping a headache, and are usually used in older children and teenagers. However, they can give people a very relaxing "buzz," and can be addictive. Use should therefore be limited and strictly supervised. Other side effects include sleepiness and dizziness, and the potential for rebound headaches.

Midrin. Midrin is a combination of three compounds: isometheptene mucate (which constricts blood vessels), acetaminophen, and dichloralphenazone (a sedative). While it can stop mild-to-moderate migraine attacks and tension headaches, it can be a hard medication for children to swallow because it comes in the form of large capsules. Dizziness, sleepiness, and stomach upset are the most common side effects.

Triptans. Triptan medications are the latest, and probably the greatest, treatment for migraine. There are several different medications available. Sumatriptan (Imitrex) was the first to come out, and has pill, nasal spray, and injectable dosing methods. As of this writing, the company that makes Imitrex is trying to obtain FDA approval to treat children. Rizatriptan (Maxalt) is available in pills that can either be swallowed or that melt quickly in your mouth. Naratriptan (Amerge) and zolmitriptan (Zomig) are available as pills, and Zomig makes a "meltaway" tablet as well. Injectable sumatriptan may be helpful in the treatment of cluster headaches, because it works the fastest.

All of these medications affect serotonin receptors and work in several different ways, including blood vessel constriction. They work fairly quickly, getting rid of headaches within an hour or two. They all have similar side effects: a potential feeling of burning or tightening of the face, neck, and chest, as well as sleepiness, dizziness, or nausea. However, these side effects tend to be minor and the medications are generally very effective.

Although these medications all seem to work the same way, some may work better for your child than others. Some may work a little quicker, some may last a little longer, some may have fewer side effects than others for your child. They should not be given on the same day as other vasoconstrictors like ergotamine medications, and they can lead to rebound headaches if taken too often.

Steroids. Steroid medications such as Prednisone are used to treat severe headaches, or headaches that stick around for a long time and don't respond to other treatments. They are often used to stop severe migraines or bouts of cluster headaches. Steroids are anti-inflammatory medications, and they are especially useful in children who should not receive vasoconstrictors (children with certain types of heart disease; children who have had strokes; and children whose headaches are associated with numbness, weakness, or prolonged auras, for example). They are usually given over the course of several days, starting with a high dose and tapering to a lower dose.

Steroids can have a lot of side effects. They can have effects on mood, making children quite hyperactive. They can cause children to eat a lot and have difficulty sleeping. If used for a long time, they can depress a child's immune response.

Anti-emetics. A lot of children throw up frequently and repeatedly during a migraine attack, and medications that treat nausea and vomiting are particularly helpful for them (and their parents). There are several different kinds, marketed under the trade names Tigan, Compazine, and Phenergan. Most come in a suppository form as well as a pill or liquid form.

Sleepiness is the most common side effect. However, unusual side effects called extrapyramidal reactions can be seen with some anti-emetic medications. These reactions range from stiffness to jitteriness to unusual movements of the mouth called tardive dyskinesia. Side effects like this are more common in children than adults.

What medication can I give my child if he is throwing up?

Throwing up is a very common symptom associated with migraines, and it happens more with children than with adults (the reasons behind this are unclear). When a child is vomiting, it's hard for a parent to get them to swallow a medication. This can lead to the child being more upset, crying, and throwing up even more as the parent is trying to get him to swallow the medicine. Furthermore, even if the parent can get the child to swallow the medication, the child may quickly throw it up again. Parents may have trouble knowing how much of the medication was actually absorbed before the child threw it up.

Luckily, there are a variety of alternate ways for a child to take medicine, and these methods do not require the cooperation of the child's mouth or stomach. The standard alternate routes have been either rectal administration by suppository form or injections of medication into a child's vein or muscles (the latter is usually done for severely affected children in the context of an emergency room visit). However, in the past five to ten years, more pleasant alternatives have been developed. Several medications such as sumatriptan (Imitrex) are available in a nasal spray, and others such as rizatriptan (Maxalt) are available in a tablet that immediately dissolves in the child's mouth.

Very young children (under six years old), who are the most likely to have headaches dominated by vomiting, will still probably use the anti-emetics that are delivered by suppository. They have been used for a long time in these situations, and are generally quite safe. Older children may be best served by the newer preparations (although many are not FDA approved for them), which they can administer themselves. The nasal sprays are easy for a child to use. The child's head should be tilted forward for best absorption. The "melt-in-your-mouth" medications are generally perceived by children to be "cool" and are almost foolproof to use. The pill is opened directly into the child's mouth, then it melts right away. Children generally approve of the taste, and no water or other liquid is required to wash it down. It can be a very convenient way of taking medication in situations where a migraine with vomiting is provoked by car travel (or other situations where a drink may not be handy).

It is important, though, to encourage the child to drink something after the vomiting has calmed down a bit. Children, with their small body size, can get dehydrated quickly. If your child has just been through a bout of vomiting, try to rehydrate him slowly and steadily, possibly by using sips of sugar- and salt-containing fluids like Gatorade or Pedialyte.

TREATMENT OF INTRACTABLE HEADACHES

Some children can have headaches that go on for weeks or months at a time, every day, all the time. These usually start gradually and build up over a few days or so, but they may start intensely and just stay that way. Some children seem to be more prone to these than others; they seldom get short headaches and usually get these long ones. Other children never get these. Intractable headaches seem to be more common in teenagers than in younger children. Different factors can contribute: some are thought to be a form of a migraine (an intractable migraine is also called a status migrainosus, or migraine status), some are thought to start out as tension-type headaches, and some may be due to overuse of medication (rebound headaches) or constant stress. Intractable headaches can be enormously difficult on a family, and they are discussed further in Chapter 7.

Treatment of these headaches can be quite difficult and needs to be individually tailored to the particular child. Medication overuse needs to be looked into as the first step, because it is so common. Psychological factors such as stress can also contribute. The psychological causes of the pain need to be considered in all of these long headaches—stress may be an explanation for why the headache started, or the stress from the long-term headache may actually have compounded the existing stress in the child's life.

During a long headache, many different medications are usually used. If this is the first time a child has experienced such a headache, his parent will probably give him some sort of over-the-counter medication (such as acetaminophen or ibuprofen) when he first complains of head pain. When this is not effective, the child is brought to the doctor. The doctor may have the child try Midrin, one of the triptan medications, ergot medications, or the other medications for the treatment of headache listed above. But what if those don't work? (And the longer the headache has gone on by the time these are tried, the less likely they are to work.)

At this point, the child may need a specialist. The specialist may try intravenous treatments like dihydroergotamine (DHE) or steroids like Prednisone. He may also start the child on one of the preventative medications for headache discussed in this chapter. These medications can be helpful in turning around a long headache, and a family who is suffering through a long headache will generally desire as much prevention of similar symptoms in the future as possible.

In general, the more medications that have been used and found ineffective, the less likely it will be that somebody will find a "magic bullet" that will end the headache. Of course, the medications will need to be reviewed to make sure that the child has taken them in proper doses, and that they have been given adequate time in which to work. However, if the child just doesn't seem to be responding to any medications, alternative strategies such as biobehavioral training may be helpful (see Chapter 5).

DRUG INTERACTIONS

Specific potential drug interactions should be discussed with your child's doctor, but there are some general categories of interactions to be aware of.

The triptan medications (Imitrex, Maxalt, Amerge, and Zomig) can interact with several types of medications. They may interact with some of the beta-blockers, especially propranolol (Inderal), raising the level of triptan medication in the blood. They should not be used with a class of medications called monoamine oxidase inhibitors (MAOIs), which are used to treat certain psychiatric disorders and are rarely prescribed for children.

In general, drugs that cause constriction of blood vessels should probably not be used together. Specific mechanisms of actions of the different drugs are discussed earlier in the chapter, but for example triptans and ergotamines both work that way. They should not be given at the same time; if your child is going to try both medications, there should be about a day's space in between.

Herbal remedies do need to be discussed with your doctor, because some of them may interact with conventional medications. Information on herbal medications is much more limited, but for example St. John's Wort has been shown to affect liver enzymes, which are responsible for metabolizing other medications you might take.

On the whole, all of these medications can be taken with food and with over-the-counter cold medications.

CHAPTER 5

Take a Massage and Call Me in the Morning
Nondrug Therapies

I have been trained in traditional medicine, but believe in the value of some nontraditional treatments to prevent and treat headaches. I do not believe in the value of every nontraditional method, however (just as I do not believe in the value of every traditional method). This chapter will focus on the nontraditional methods that have some common sense behind them, some proof that they work, or at least have the benefit of being inexpensive or practical to try—and those that are fairly certain to be harmless. Remember, there are hundreds of ways to treat headaches. No single practitioner is going to be able to guide you through them all, nor should he or she even attempt to do so. Try the remedies that best fit you and your child.

DIETARY INTERVENTIONS

As explained more fully in Chapter 2, the relationship between migraines and particular foods has been studied much more thoroughly in adults than in children. Therefore, dietary recommendations to prevent headaches from occurring are generally more easy to make in adults than in children. To briefly review, examples of some of the most common food triggers for adults include yellow cheeses (like cheddar), red wine, MSG, nitrates, and aspartame. The idea behind dietary interventions is to identify dietary triggers for headaches and try to avoid them.

So, what's a parent to do? You could analyze every gram of food that goes into your child's body, or you could give up before you even start. Like the rest of the advice in this book, my approach tends to be more middle-of-the-road, focusing on what is practical and what makes common sense for you and your child.

If headache frequency is less than "all the time" or "every day," it makes sense to keep track of the foods that your child is eating on the days she is having headaches. If headaches are coming every day, one is less likely to uncover a pattern of food triggers unless the same foods happen to be consumed every day. Parents can keep track of eating and headache patterns in a "headache diary."

HOW TO MAKE A HEADACHE DIARY

Physicians frequently ask parents to make a headache diary without getting into specifics of what it should consist of or how it should be made. The variety of triggers that such diaries reveal is quite wide, and a headache diary may also give physicians a clue as to how seriously the patient and family view the problem of the headaches. Remember that the exact form of the diary isn't as important as the information contained in it. Here are some helpful tips:

- *Write legibly...* Although this may sound ironic coming from a doctor, what we can't read we can't help you interpret. Especially with busy primary care physicians, the time you will have available to discuss your diary with your doctor is going to be limited, so make your diary as neat as possible.
- *But use whatever form you want.* It doesn't matter whether information is recorded on a computer, loose paper, or a calendar. Use what is easily accessible to you and your child. Remember, though, that keeping track of the calendar dates when the headaches occurred is important, espe-

cially for girls, whose headaches may be related to their monthly cycle.

- *Focus on basic information...* While it would not be impossible to write down everything your child was exposed to every day, it certainly would be a daunting task. Focus on the days where the headaches occur.
- *But be complete.* Write down activities that occurred on those days, foods and drinks ingested, and any potentially stressful occurrences or worries that your child may have had. Pay particular attention to the hours before the headache started. Record what days the headaches occurred, what your child was doing when they started, how long they lasted, what your child took for them, and what activities your child did after they started. (Did your child go to bed? Play? Miss school or homework?)

The diary should be kept until you start to see definite improvement in your child's symptoms. A sample form of a headache diary can be found in Appendix A.

If the same foods start showing up in conjunction with the headaches, it would be reasonable to try to eliminate those foods from the diet and look to see whether the child's headache frequency goes down. The pattern of when your child eats may be important, too. Some headaches are triggered by hunger or thirst, so if your child is eating later than normal when headaches occur, providing him with a small snack might be enough to ward off some or all of the headaches.

Consider also any new eating or drinking patterns that may have started when headaches started to worsen. One common issue here is caffeine. For many people caffeine will help get rid of a headache. This is thought to be due to caffeine's ability to constrict blood vessels, and indeed caffeine is a frequently found ingredient in compound headache medications (see Chapter 4). However, other people can be quite sensitive to the effects of caffeine, in which case even slight variations in the amount they consume can lead to "rebound headaches." Rebound headaches result when the usual amount of dietary caffeine decreases a little; one theory is that there is rebound dilatation of the blood vessels of the head, triggering what can be a very painful headache. Remember that caffeine comes not only in food and drink but also in over-the-counter pain relievers such as Excedrin Migraine, so look at all the sources your child may be consuming. Sources of caffeine include coffee (remember to include lattes, espresso, etc.), certain teas, chocolate, sodas, and a variety of medications and other supplements (some over-the-counter cold remedies, pain relievers, diet supplements, diuretics, and "energy formulas"). Has your child recently been using stimulants like No-Doz to cram for tests? These stimulants are loaded with caffeine.

ISSUES TO CONSIDER IN FORMING A DIETARY TREATMENT FOR HEADACHES

While it is always worthwhile to consider whether certain foods are triggering headaches in your child, it is not always easy to make the interventions. While most children will understand that eating a certain food will make them sick and translate that into the behavior of avoiding a particular food, others simply will not modify their eating habits. Worse still, others will turn that knowledge into a control issue between parent and child—a child's way to develop a sense of independence by defying a parent's rules and wishes. There are other issues to consider too: when to relax the rules, and what to do when there is a clash with other eating issues.

Here are some of the major issues to consider when developing a dietary program to help with your child's headaches:

- *The age of your child.* The easiest age to control your child's diet is when your child is quite small—in the preschool years. School-age children are more influenced by peers about what to eat. Preschool has its own challenges, too, as a child may have intense food preferences during those years, but at least you have control over the choices he has available. So when trying to come up with a food program for your child, know that one really has to educate older children about how to choose for themselves when you are not there to choose for them.

- *The temperament of your child.* The argument follows similar lines as those stated above. Oppositional children will not follow a diet that you set for them and will break a diet willfully, despite the raging headache that may follow. The best way to avoid this problem is to have your child involved in designing the diet, and if it is broken not to punish them directly—just point out that the headache that follows is of their doing, a consequence of their own actions. Eventually, they will either decide to follow the diet or not, but it will not become a control issue between you and your child.
- *Special occasions.* Times will come up when your child will be forced into the decision (or you will be forced to decide for him): does he eat the chocolate birthday cake that every one else at the party is eating (even though he will pay for it later), or does he refuse? The issue here is that you really want your child to feel like a normal kid and not have to go to extremes to prevent headaches. How do you help your child make these choices? It really depends on the severity of the headaches, and how certain they are to occur following ingestion of the foods. If you know that your child will definitely be emergency-room material if he takes even one bite, I'd strongly encourage him to refuse. If, however, he might get a mild headache by eating it, let him do so if he so wishes.
- *Other eating issues.* Eating disorders such as anorexia and bulimia are on the rise in this country, especially in females.

There is absolutely no reason to suspect that following a special diet to prevent migraines would in any way contribute to the development of any sort of eating disorder. However, it may be that your child with migraines also has an eating disorder (or a tendency towards an eating disorder); in this case, you should not focus on food as a source of headaches.

- *Be low-key, and don't eliminate foods unless you are sure.* Some children may become anxious when you are in the process of figuring out the food triggers. As they see you trying to "pin" the headaches on different foods, they may become anxious about those particular foods: "It might cause me to have headaches, what should I do?" They may become worried when they eat those foods, and the worry can itself generate a headache. The longer this goes on, the better the chance that a child could develop more distress about more and more foods.

ENVIRONMENTAL MANIPULATIONS

Recently the issue of sensitivities or allergies to a variety of environmental exposures has been given a lot of press. We are surrounded on a daily basis by hundreds of thousands of different chemicals, some of which are natural and some of which are man-made. The man-made chemicals were generally developed for a purpose (cleaning houses or bodies, getting rid of insects, and fertilizing soil, just to name a few), but some people may suffer unintended consequences because of the way their immune systems react to them. For some people, one of the consequences could be headaches.

Just as sorting out dietary triggers (which really could be thought of as a form of environmental allergy) can be quite complicated, sorting out environmental triggers is even more complex. At least with dietary triggers you can write down what you ate; environmental exposures are much less visible. You can smell them and touch them without even thinking of them (just consider the number of cosmetics and personal hygiene products that a person is exposed to every day). For some, certain environmental lighting patterns (such as fluorescent lights) or noises (particularly loud noises) are clear triggers. Again, what's a parent to do? Place the child in an allergen-free bubble to get rid of headaches?

The approach needs to involve practical common sense. Parents can use a headache diary to consider common triggers, and then try to avoid them as much as possible. The most common triggers include loud noises and bright lights, and parents can use earplugs and sunglasses to try to mitigate their effects. Another important trigger is cigarette smoking. Children who are themselves smoking, and those children who are exposed to cigarette smoke via second-hand smoking, are exposing themselves to substances that are very potent headache triggers. Both the nicotine and the carbon monoxide in the cigarettes affect blood vessel size, constricting and expanding them respectively. Studies have shown that the more you smoke and the more nicotine you are exposed to, the worse your headaches are likely to be. If your child has chronic headaches and smokes at all or is exposed to smoke, the very first intervention with a likely positive effect would be to stop exposure to smoke.

Again, be low-key in your efforts and try not to generate too much anxiety for your child. You don't want him to begin to believe that everything around him is dangerous.

HERBAL SUPPLEMENTS

Herbal medicine focuses on plant sources for medicinal purposes. A variety of herbs are used and are bought over-the-counter without a prescription in a variety of drugstores and health food stores. Many areas around the world use herbs to treat a variety of conditions; further, in western medical practices, a number of common medications are based upon these naturally-occurring compounds.

What could be wrong with taking herbs? Just like everything found naturally, some herbs are good for you, and some are potentially harmful. Furthermore, just as with conventional medications, side effects are a potential problem. However, unlike conventional medications, the FDA does not test or put the herbs through an approval process. Since just one conventional medication in thirteen makes it through the rigorous testing demanded by the FDA (which proves efficacy and delineates the most common side effects), I do wonder how many herbs are being used out there that really should be "weeded out" (no pun intended). There have been recent articles in the press about the increasing practice of giving children herbal supplements, without the experience or data to justify doing so. Also, there is no universal standard of purity. This means that what is listed on the bottle may or may not be present in the pill, or it may be present at a very low concentration. Furthermore, the pill is not guaranteed to dissolve once swallowed, and the contents of the pill must be absorbed for it to have any effect!

Caveats aside, some herbs probably are of benefit to some people with headaches. The most common herb used is feverfew. Feverfew is used both to stop acute migraine attacks in progress as well as on a daily basis as a preventative measure. It is usually prescribed in liquid form and given at a drops-per-hour or drops-per-day rate. It seems to have very few side effects.

Other herbs used include lavender, peppermint, ginger, and chamomile in teas and compresses. Eating twelve almonds (which contain a natural form of aspirin) has been a common folk remedy in Africa and Asia. Taking a spoonful of honey, or honey mixed with apple cider vinegar, has also been used.

Homeopathy is a type of herbal medicine that uses highly diluted concentrations of herbs and other substances. The substances can be diluted so much that there is no trace of them in the final product. The idea behind homeopathy is to use these substances to stimulate the body to heal itself. Homeopathy is very widely used throughout the world, although many medical professionals (myself included) trained in the use of conventional medication are skeptical that the homeopathic medications themselves are actually providing relief. There is a concept called "the placebo effect" that may apply: If one believes that a remedy will work, even taking a sugar pill may be curative for a variety of conditions.

Herbal and homeopathic medication are often administered under the guidance of a naturopath, who has learned about these substances in a specialized training program.

VITAMIN SUPPLEMENTS: RIBOFLAVIN AND MAGNESIUM

We are a nation that takes a great many supplements of vitamins and minerals. Many Americans swallow a multivitamin daily, and others take megadoses of certain selected vitamins or minerals. What is safe and what is not, what is beneficial and what is not, still needs to be worked out in greater detail. The Nobel-winning scientist Linus Pauling championed megadoses of vitamin C and lived to be 93. However, a recent study suggested that high doses of vitamin C lead to premature heart disease. High doses of fat-soluble vitamins (such as vitamins A and E) are known to have some toxicity. For example, too much vitamin A at certain times during pregnancy is known to cause birth defects. However, high doses of vitamin E may be protective for and effective against Alzheimer's disease. Also in question is whether the manufactured vitamin product, which isolates one or a few substances, is as protective against disease as the natural substance that the vitamin is derived from. Is taking an "antioxidant pill" as effective as eating fruits and vegetables?

Thus, like the herbal supplements described above, vitamin supplements are best taken with the figurative grain of salt. Probably the safest thing to do is to avoid megadoses of them all (megadoses being defined as multiple times the RDA, which stands for the recommended daily allowance) and to eat a healthy, well-balanced, and varied diet. If you do choose to supplement your child's diet with vitamins or minerals, look for the bottles marked with the USP insignia. USP stands for United States Pharmacopoeia. It is an assurance that there is a standard amount of the compound in the pills and that the pills are guaranteed to dissolve and deliver the product to your child's body.

There are two substances in particular that have been shown in a few studies to have some benefit. Riboflavin (also known as vitamin B2) has, in at least two studies in respected medical journals, been shown to have some benefits for adult migraine sufferers. Given at doses of 400 mg per day over a period of months, both the frequency and severity of migraine headaches lessened for more than half the adults who took them. Side effects at those doses were minimal; mild diarrhea and frequent urination were seen in a few patients. Teenagers could probably take the same doses with similar side effects (although the effectiveness may or may not be as high). However, in trying to extrapolate and use these results for younger children, there are some practical problems involved. It is unclear what dose to use and whether children would suffer similar side effects. Also, most stores carry riboflavin in 50 mg supplements. To take 400 mg would require a child to swallow eight pills (on a daily basis). When this is taken into consideration, most parents seriously consider other options. (The most common response is, "You try giving that to him!")

Magnesium, which is a mineral, may also be helpful with regard to headache prevention and treatment. The daily intake of magnesium has decreased over the past century. Magnesium has been implicated in affecting the tone of blood vessels, and in this way it may have some relationship to headache genesis or treatment. It has been suggested that some migraine patients may benefit from magnesium supplementation, especially those with menstrual-related migraines, but it has not really been established whether (or how) this works.

ACUPUNCTURE

Acupuncture has been in continuous use for more than three thousand years, originating in China. The idea behind acupuncture is that it treats imbalances in the energy (called *chi*) flowing throughout the body. There are thought to be twelve major pathways that the energy flows along; energy could either be too low or excessive. The head holds a special role, as it is a central meeting place of a number of energy channels, and where in the head the pain is located may indicate to the practitioner what the source is. This leads to various kinds of treatment, from adjusting the diet to the more-familiar acupuncture needles. These are very thin needles inserted in selected areas, left in place for minutes at a time. The needles are thought to enhance energy flow. It may take several sessions to see an effect.

Of all alternative treatments, acupuncture is one of the most respected in conventional circles because of its perceived effectiveness. There is very little information available for children, however. Parents usually ask whether the child will tolerate the needles. A recent study that dealt mostly with teenage children reported that acupuncture was safe, pleasant, and helpful. What of the younger children, however? Although some will not tolerate the treatments, a two-year-old patient of mine went to an acupuncturist who was comfortable with children, and she did very well. When children are given the choice between acupuncture and biofeedback as alternative therapies, though, many will try the biofeedback first when they hear about the needles!

I would recommend trying acupuncture for children whose parents want to avoid traditional medicines, for children who are too young to try biofeedback (generally, ten years or younger), or for older children if they would like to try it. When looking for an acupuncturist, parents should make sure the needles are sterilized and disposed of after just one use (otherwise, they could carry infectious disease like HIV or herpes). It is important, too, to find an acupuncturist who is comfortable with treating children of your child's age.

ACUPRESSURE

Acupressure is an ancient technique that may give some relief to children with headaches. It is probably most effective as part of an overall relaxation program designed to be used at the onset of a headache before it gets too severe. If it isn't used right away, chances are it will be less effective. There is very little evidence to say that acupressure works in children, but as it doesn't have any side effects, it is probably worth a try in some. A child five years of age or older can be trained to do these techniques to some degree. The older children may be trained to associate relaxation breathing with the acupressure techniques, thus maximizing their effectiveness.

The idea behind acupressure is that firm pressure on certain body points can alleviate a variety of symptoms including several types of headaches. Here are several points associated with the head:

- Pressure midway between the eyebrows
- Pressure on the upper eyesockets, where the eyebrow meets the nose
- Pressure in the back of the head, in the center just underneath the base of the skull
- Pressure on both outer sides of the vertical neck muscles just underneath the base of the skull.

Although not a formal acupressure technique, some people do get relief simply by tying a tight band around the forehead.

BIOFEEDBACK AND BIOBEHAVIORAL TRAINING

Biofeedback (ideally, *biobehavioral training*, which not only encompasses biofeedback but also a number of behavioral interventions) is one of the most powerful tools in the arsenal against headaches. The idea behind it is to use the power of the mind to influence the body, without the use of drugs. It has been popular for approximately fifteen years as a way to treat children who suffer from chronic headaches. The "biofeedback" part of this therapy is where the children can be trained to alter skin temperature, muscle tension, and even heart rate and brain rhythms. In the best of circumstances biofeedback is only part of an overall behavioral program called biobehavioral training. This type of program has proven effectiveness in both adults and children, and it has greatly helped a number of my patients.

Biobehavioral training involves a number of sessions, typically ten to twelve, so the parents and the child have to be willing to devote the time and energy needed. It is crucial for the parents to believe that this type of training will work and that for their child, medications may not be the answer. If the parents do not have an attitude of acceptance toward this method but instead believe that their child just hasn't found the right medication, or that a medical diagnosis may have been missed, the child will not do well in biobehavioral training.

During the sessions, a variety of techniques will be used to teach the child to modify the usual responses of his body to stress and pain. There are two major goals. One is to stop small headaches that may occur from becoming large headaches that interfere with normal daily life. The second goal is to try to alter behavior patterns that may be contributing to the headaches.

The specific methods used vary from program to program, but keeping a headache diary may be involved. This diary may provide clues to behavioral patterns that are involved with your child's headaches; modifying those behavioral patterns can improve the headaches. For example, you and your child may note that the headaches occur when your child is worried about something; seeing such a pattern may suggest that your child needs help with stress management rather than looking to medications. You may also see that your child is getting out of schoolwork or chores on a regular basis because of these headaches, which most children view as a benefit. You need to think about what role this benefit may be playing in your child's headaches. Most children at one point or other will pretend to be sick specifically in order to avoid something they do not want to do, like go to school. In that case, the endpoint (avoiding school, whatever it may be) is called "primary gain." In most children with chronic headache, however, the situation is not as simple. They do not have the headache in the first place in order to avoid a particular situation, but they do note subconsciously that when they have a headache they stay home and mom or dad fusses over them and gives them special attention. These subconscious benefits, called "secondary gains," are important, because they can influence both the frequency and severity of headaches. Remember, pain is quite subjective; there is no way to tell exactly how much a headache is hurting your child except by your child's behavior (see Chapter 1). Your child's pain behavior may become exaggerated (consciously or subconsciously) as a result of secondary gain, and the diary may help you think about what secondary gains are involved.

Once patterns of behavior are identified, how do the biobehavioral techniques modify them? Again, different programs may involve different techniques, but your child should be taught how to relax his body when a headache starts. The child can then use the relaxation techniques when he feels a headache coming on to abort the headache. Biofeedback training, in which normal body functions are modified by focusing on them mentally, is used as an aid to help teach a child how to relax his body and change normal body functions associated with stress.

For example, one biofeedback technique involves an instrument for electromyography (EMG) to help teach a child how to relax muscles he may be tensing as a headache is coming on, or during the headache. The EMG machine uses a thin needle to transmit electricity to a central processor, which then causes loud sounds to be emitted when muscles are tense. The patient uses the audible feedback from the EMG to relax his muscles; when his muscles are truly relaxed, there will be silence from the EMG. (This technique is not just for tension-type headaches. Migraines and other headaches involve muscle tension to the same degree; see Chapter 2.)

Another biofeedback technique involves changes in body temperature. In stressful situations and during headaches, people's hands tend to become cold. With temperature monitors on their hand, children can actually be trained to modify blood flow, warming their hands. By doing so, they tend to relax and improve their headaches. Some programs may also use an electroencephalogram (EEG) that monitors brain waves with electrodes placed on the scalp; others may train your child to focus on heart rate. When your child can get his body to respond, that feeling may be combined with visual imagery techniques (where your child pictures situations that are relaxing for him) or breathing exercises. The overall goal is that, away from the monitors and during a time when a headache is building, your child can start visualizing or breathing in a very relaxing way and focus on feeling his body loosen up.

The above biofeedback techniques let your child know, in a very concrete way, how his body responds to stress. When your child knows that he can control these functions, you are giving him a powerful tool that he may not have had before: a feeling of control over his body. Children who have chronic headaches tend to feel helpless and at the mercy of the headaches, and it has been shown that getting a sense of control over pain may very well improve how a child responds to it.

Such programs may also give your child some other types of mental strategies to use when a headache is coming on. A child with recurrent headaches may think of himself as abnormal, sick, or worthless, and these negative thoughts may cause his headache to worsen. Giving your child positive thoughts to think about, or at least stopping the negative self-thoughts, can be quite beneficial. Your child may be taught to think of something simple over and over again: "I'm OK, I'm OK, I'm OK."

To participate in a biobehavioral program, a child has to be old enough to really concentrate well. He has to be able to understand the training techniques being used and to take the initiative to use them independently. He must also believe in and be willing to participate in the training. Most of the time, children under the age of eight will not have the maturity to participate effectively in this sort of training program. Adolescents, though, can benefit tremendously from biobehavioral programs, as they tend to have stress-related headaches and also tend to have a natural focus on their bodies. Simple migraine headaches (those not complicated by severe vomiting, visual, sensory, or motor changes) seem to respond best, and the technique is of particular use for those children who have frequent or daily headaches. Biobehavioral training, if done properly, can be a wonderful stress management technique, giving a child a tool that can be beneficial over a lifetime in many different situations. And of course, except for the time involved, there are no side effects!

There are quite a few practitioners of biofeedback out there; how do you, as a parent, select the one that is right for your child? Probably the best is to ask your child's doctor for a referral to a practitioner who they think has a good track record in working with children. Your local hospital, especially one with a large pediatric department, may be another source. If you are looking for a practitioner on your own, make sure of the following aspects: First, look for one who has experience in treating children. Also, as biofeedback is being used for a number of medical conditions, look for a practitioner who specializes in headaches. Finally, if EMG needles are being used, make sure that they are presterilized and disposed of after just one use. Like acupuncture needles, EMG needles could be a potential source of infectious disease.

AROMATHERAPY

Aromatherapy uses extracts from plants to treat a variety of conditions, including headaches. The "essential oils" are rubbed on, inhaled, bathed in, or pressed on by compresses (but not taken by mouth). While I am skeptical of the ability of the plants themselves to cure the underlying cause of the headache, I am confident of the ability of soothing smells to help promote relaxation—and the relaxation itself may then lead to healing. Therefore, the specific type of oil or method used does not seem to me to be the most important factor. If you want to try this method, choose an oil that your child likes (such as peppermint, rosemary, lemon, or lavender) and a delivery system that your child will enjoy and find relaxing. For example, if your child likes to bathe, add some of the oil to the bathwater. If your child is old enough to cooperate with a facial steam, pour some boiling water into a large bowl, add some oil, and cover your child's head and the bowl with a large towel. Have your child inhale deeply for as long as the steam is rising. Because of the risk of hot water burns, supervise carefully and only try this with a child who is old enough to understand the directions well (probably eight years and older).

TEMPERATURE MANIPULATIONS: HOT OR COLD?

Many patients with migraine feel that simply putting a hot or a cold washcloth on their forehead makes them feel better. Some people respond best to ice or other cold substances; others feel that heat is much more helpful. Whatever your child responds best to is what should be used. There is no medical reason to choose one over the other. A number of commercial heat or cold packs are available, but a hot or cold towel works just as well for many.

EXERCISE

In my opinion, the value of exercise with regard to headache prevention has been quite underestimated in traditional medicine. Children need regular exercise for a variety of reasons, and more and more of them are not getting enough of it. Fear of playing outside (because of medical concerns like asthma or pollution, or social concerns like kidnapping or other dangers), organized after-school activities that take up a great deal of time, and of course the seduction of TV and computer games all contribute to a population of children who are growing more obese and further out of shape. In addition, childhood exercise today seems to be taking a more organized and formal form, such as playing on teams in organized sports situations. This often takes out the more imaginative and free play elements that used to occur more regularly when a group of kids could roam over the neighborhood for hours playing at whatever came into their heads.

Ideally, exercise should involve both elements of aerobic stimulation—pushing your body to achieve an elevated heart rate and maintaining that heart rate for at least twenty to thirty minutes at a time—and imaginative fun. Both aspects add to a sense of satisfaction, accomplishment, and well-being that contributes to overall good health and an improved mental outlook.

If you live in the type of neighborhood where kids can safely bike, climb trees, or just run around together, great. This "natural exercise" will just be viewed as plain fun by the children. (In contrast, I think of my days jogging, which I did not particularly enjoy but rather viewed simply as an efficient way to exercise—it was more of a chore than something to be enjoyed.) Try to find an activity that your child really likes and that sneaks in exercise at the same time. Got a budding tap dancer? A martial artist just waiting to chop his way out? It doesn't matter what the activity is, as long as it is done and enjoyed!

Yoga can have great benefits with regard to headache treatment and prevention. However, only older teenagers will probably be able to have the maturity and concentration needed to participate effectively in this combination of stretching, postural exercises, breathing, and meditative techniques.

Where should all of this wonderful exercising be done? Again, do the best you can, but try to get your child outdoors for at least some time every day. There's no concrete proof that fresh air is the best—but it's hard to argue that it isn't!

CHIROPRACTIC MANIPULATIONS AND PHYSICAL THERAPY

Chiropractors are treating increasing numbers of children, as the amount of interest in alternative medicine grows. Chiropractors focus on the spinal column and musculoskeletal structure. Chiropractors believe that headaches come from a misalignment of the spine or spinal muscles, and that by realigning the imbalance the headaches will be improved. They may take X rays and use a variety of techniques to manipulate the vertebral column. These techniques may involve stretching, quick jerks (also known as "cracking"), and deep tissue massage.

Physical therapists may use some similar techniques, but the focus is less on the spine and more on overall muscle use. They may do a combination of massage therapy, electrical stimulation, and traction exercises. There are more specific techniques such as craniosacral therapy that are available.

Many people have had good experiences with their chiropractors and physical therapists, and the techniques can be quite helpful. I would caution against the use of "cracking," especially in the neck area. There are important blood vessels going to the brain that run through the upper cervical vertebrae in the neck, and these could potentially be injured by certain maneuvers. Although most chiropractors I've talked to say their techniques prevent such things from happening, I've seen patients who have had medical problems from them.

Like all therapies used, give your chiropractor some time to cure your child's headaches, and if you are not achieving the desired result, consider other treatments (or look again at the potential causes of the headaches). Again, in selecting a chiropractor, look for one who has a lot of experience in treating both children and headaches. A chiropractor who does not have such experience may not help your child and may not be sensitive to differences between a child's and an adult's musculoskeletal physiology. Children's bones and muscles, especially during phases of active growth, are different from those of adults.

CHAPTER 6

A Doctor's Visit

How a Doctor Thinks About Your Child's Headache

Even young children want to know what will happen when they go to the doctor. Mostly, they want to know "will it hurt?" and "will I have to get a shot?" Many parents who are used to taking their children to the pediatrician just for regular check-ups don't know how to answer those questions when it comes to a specific doctor's visit about headaches. What does a visit to a doctor for headaches involve? This chapter will take you through a typical medical evaluation for headaches, explaining what might happen in the doctor's office. Reading this section will help you to prepare your child in advance for the visit, which will generally make the visit more productive. A child who knows what to expect is less likely to be fearful and more likely to participate in the experience, and that will help your doctor a great deal. You can also use this section to help understand how a doctor thinks about headaches, which will help you to ask appropriate questions. Knowing what should happen will also help you to evaluate how thorough your doctor is being. However, remember that the information discussed in this chapter is very detailed. Your child's doctor may not need to go through it all in order to come up with the correct diagnosis.

• • •

Every doctor has his or her own style, of course, but all doctor visits share a common structure composed of four sections.

First, questions will be asked, both of the parents and of the child (depending on the child's age, of course). Some doctors have a "Headache Questionnaire" that you will fill out in the waiting room or the exam room before you see the doctor, but this should be followed up with more detailed questions that you and your child will answer in person. This part of the evaluation is called the "history" section, and it is of great importance in the evaluation of headaches. Next, the doctor will examine your child. The physical examination will be of your child's whole body, but will focus on a neurologic examination. Third, your doctor will consider the information gathered in the history and the physical examination, and come up with a list of reasons (presumptive diagnoses) that could explain why your child has a headache. Finally, the doctor will go down the list to decide if further tests are needed and what treatment is correct.

QUESTIONS YOUR DOCTOR SHOULD ASK

Your doctor should ask a lot of questions about the headaches, because the answers to those questions are very important in determining the headaches' cause! A good detective might be able to solve a mystery just by hearing about a crime, without personally seeing a single shred of evidence. Similarly, a good doctor can often determine the cause of the headache on the basis of the history alone. As a matter of fact, how a doctor thinks about a headache can be pretty similar to how a detective solves a mystery. A detective should ask enough questions so that he can visualize himself at the scene, and the doctor should ask enough questions so that he really gets an idea of what the patient is experiencing.

How can you help your doctor?

- Think about the questions in this chapter in advance.

- Try to write down the answers to some of the questions ahead of time in an organized fashion.
- Talk about the questions with your child before seeing the doctor. This is most important with children who are less verbal or who may be scared during the exam time.
- Talk to family members in advance in order to get an accurate family medical history.
- If your child is in school or daycare, you may also wish to speak to his teachers about what they have observed.

Your doctor will need a lot of information! Here are some questions you might be asked and the reasons behind the questions.

How frequent are the headaches? Every day? Every two weeks? Once every few months? Think about whether they are getting more frequent, less frequent, or have remained stable over time. Headaches that are stable or are actually improving will probably mean that fewer tests need to be done. If a headache is happening frequently enough, your doctor will probably need to focus on preventative strategies for the headache (see Chapter 3). Headaches that are getting more frequent may mean that obtaining a diagnosis and initiating treatment needs to happen quickly.

Are there situations that can trigger a headache? Some people have headaches triggered by certain foods. Others find that being hungry or thirsty can trigger a headache. Stress usually increases the frequency of headaches, but not always. Some patients get headaches at a particular time of day, or at a particular time of a monthly menstrual cycle. Sometimes exercise provokes them. Paying attention to the pattern of headaches will help your doctor both diagnose the cause of the headaches as well as to manage them. There are some worrisome patterns, and there are some that are not so bad. An example of a worrisome pattern would be headaches that wake up a child in the morning and are associated with vomiting. This sort of pattern *might* increase the suspicion of a possible brain tumor (see Chapter 2). On the other hand, patterns associated with migraine include headaches triggered by certain foods, or headaches that come on a cyclical basis. Exercise-induced headaches often require diagnostic imaging studies such as CT scans or MRI (discussed later in this chapter). If triggers are known, your doctor may focus on removing some of those triggers as part of your child's treatment. If the headaches are only associated with a particular location, then environmental factors about that location (such as carbon monoxide exposure) should be reviewed and explored.

How long does the headache usually last? This can be a hard question to answer or to interpret, because medications that your child may be taking can shorten the natural length of a headache. Some headaches, such as cluster headaches or trigeminal neuralgia, typically last only a few seconds or minutes. Other headaches such as migraine tend to be longer, often lasting hours or even days.

Overall, are the headaches getting better or worse? Usually, when a headache is decreasing in frequency it is usually decreasing in severity, but not always. Overall, headaches that are gaining in either frequency or intensity require more aggressive diagnoses or treatments than ones which seem to be improving.

• • •

Now, on to more specific questions about the headaches themselves.

Where does it hurt? Your doctor will probably ask your child to point to where it hurts when she has a headache. Some children will be able to demonstrate this well, usually older school-age kids or adolescents. Younger children may have a hard time doing this. It will be harder for them to remember, during the office visit, where it was hurting when they had a headache. Also they have more difficulty localizing the actual pain. Children will often rub their head when they have a headache, so try to get an idea of where it is hurting them by watching them when they have a headache. Are they consistently rubbing just the right side? Are they rubbing the center of their forehead, or the back? One-sided headaches can often be associated with migraines, but they can also be associated with blood vessel malformations as well. Sometimes, headaches jump around from one side of the head to the other. Doctors usually feel more comfortable when they hear that. It makes a blood vessel malformation less likely, and makes migraine headaches more likely.

How does the headache feel? Throbbing? Sharp? Dull? Hot? Cold? Your doctor will probably ask your child to try to describe the headache thoroughly. Younger children especially may not be able to; it is difficult even for many adults to identify and express their pain. Migraine headaches are classically throbbing, and tension headaches dull. However, no doctor should base his or her diagnosis on this part of the description alone.

Are the headaches associated with visual changes? Visual changes are frequently seen with headaches, and there are a variety of different kinds. Many times the visual changes are much shorter than the headaches. They often precede the headache but can come during the headache or, rarely, happen on their own, and the headache can follow at an entirely different time. Most visual changes are associated with migraine headaches. Sometimes people see little sparkly lights (white lights or colored lights) dancing around. Other times, people can have blurry vision; perhaps just one or two areas in their visual field can be blurry, like what you might see looking through a camera lens that has a spot of Vaseline on it. Double vision can be associated with migraines but also with pseudotumor cerebri (see Chapter 2). Are the headaches, over time, associated with changes to your child's visual field? Your visual field is what you see: normally, you see what is in front of you plus a certain amount off to each side. Tumors, depending on where they are, can affect visual fields to different extents. Your child may not notice (or be able to tell you about) the difference, especially if it happens gradually. However, you might see him bumping into things more, or having to turn his head or hold it in unusual positions to see well.

Are the headaches associated with nausea or vomiting? If the answer to this question is yes, two major categories need to come to mind: migraines or brain tumors. Migraines are most common, and the diagnosis is usually made not just on the basis of the nausea and vomiting but also on the nausea's association with other features frequently seen in migraine headaches. Brain tumors are frequently associated with vomiting, usually in the morning. The reason for this is that in children, 70 percent of tumors occur in the back of the brain. These tumors often obstruct the outflow of fluid normally produced in the center of the brain, and when the pressure builds up it makes people throw up. It usually happens early in the morning because people have been lying horizontally in bed, without the aid of gravity to help drain the fluid. However, remember that kids in general respond to stresses of many sorts by vomiting, much more so than adults. Children who throw up during a headache may simply be responding to pain, stress, or to a general medical problem.

Are the headaches associated with sensitivity to light or sound? If the answer to this question is yes, the headache is more likely to be a migraine. However, these are not very specific indicators. With a bad headache, no matter what the cause, children might feel like lying down in a dark, quiet room.

Are the headaches associated with numbness or weakness in your child's arms or legs? With this question, the doctor is not asking about vague aching feelings or rubbery feelings in the legs, but a true loss of feeling or function. As in the previous question, a positive answer to this question could suggest migraine. A particular kind of migraine called a "complicated migraine" is defined by the appearance of neurological symptoms like numbness or weakness. It can be very frightening, because it can cause paralysis just like a stroke. However, the symptoms generally resolve entirely and are rarely permanent.

Can you rate the headache pain on a scale of 1 to 10? This is a commonly asked question, but because of problems associated with having children rate pain on any sort of a scale, I don't find this a particularly useful one (see Chapter 1). I prefer to gather this information from other types of questions.

Are there any other features associated with the headaches that we haven't talked about? If there are any things that have not been discussed that concern you, be sure to bring them up with your doctor, even if she hasn't asked this question.

• • •

Your doctor will also ask questions about your child's general medical health. Does your child have any ongoing medical problems? General medical problems such as hypothyroidism or anemia can sometimes be associated with headaches. Is your child taking any medications (many of which can cause headaches as a side effect)? Are there any recent changes in your child's health that could indicate that a new medical problem might be arising?

You will also be asked about whether there is a family history of neurologic problems, or headaches specifically. It is often helpful to ask family members in advance. Most parents will know if a relative died of a brain aneurysm, but they may not know about milder kinds of headaches suffered by family members. Both migraines and aneurysms tend to run in families. If a close family member has an aneurysm, your child will run a slightly higher-than-normal risk of having one; a propensity for migraines has a much stronger tendency to be inherited.

You may also be asked about your child's temperament. Is your child introspective and analytical, where even mild problems might bother him? Or is your child happy-go-lucky, and not easily thrown off balance emotionally? The answers to questions such as these can guide the doctor in gauging just how bad the pain is and how much it is affecting your child.

You may also be asked questions about where your child has recently traveled, and whether your child has pets at home. Why would that matter? Certain infectious diseases that can cause headaches are associated with travel to particular areas or exposure to certain animals.

There is another question that I think ranks among the most important: *How are these headaches affecting your child's life and the lives of your family members?* The answer to this question will have important ramifications on the treatment, and it can also give clues about the causes of the headaches. Do these headaches prevent your child from doing well in school? Is your child even able to go to school at all? Can your child go play soccer despite the headache? Are your child's headaches causing you to miss work or neglect other family members? Are family plans being altered because they might cause your child to have a headache? Does your child seem to enjoy the attention she gets even though the headaches are painful? Do you and your spouse share similar feelings about the headaches? Or are you and your child being resented because your spouse doesn't think they are a big deal and thinks you are "babying" the kid? The more the headaches are impacting your child's life and your family's life, the more aggressively your doctor needs to seek out the cause and provide treatment—a treatment that will let your child and your family get back in control.

What if my doctor hasn't asked these questions?

Every doctor, due to a combination of training and personality, has a different style. Some will ask all these questions and more, and some might not ask them all, or ask them in different ways. If the headaches appear to be quite minor (occurring once a year, or only causing very mild pain) your doctor probably will not ask many questions about them at all. However, if you feel like your concerns are not being met, be sure to tell the doctor. He will either have to take care of those concerns in an adequate manner, or you may need to seek a second opinion.

THE PHYSICAL

After asking all those questions, it's on to the examination portion of your evaluation. If you are seeing your primary care doctor for the headaches, he may do a different kind of examination than usual. This exam should focus more on neurologic aspects than a general exam would. This will especially be true if you are seeing a neurologist, who does specialized neurological exams routinely.

The brain is a difficult organ to examine. Unlike the skin, you can't look at it. Unlike the heart, you can't hear it. You can't even feel it. So how do you examine it? You go straight to how it works.

The brain is involved in the control of your entire body. It moves your eyes, kicks your legs, and feels and interprets the world around you. Your doctor will try to detect problems in the brain by looking for problems in how it is working. Some of the things your child may be asked to do to demonstrate how his brain is working may seem kind of silly. But there is a method to this madness, and it is explained below.

General. Does your child appear ill? Is he sitting quietly? Lying in your lap with the lights in the room off? Jumping about the room? Children are notorious for being able to appear quite well even though they may be sick, so this bit of information should be just one piece of the puzzle.

Skin. The skin and the brain are formed from some of the same embryological elements, so sometimes diseases of the nervous system that can cause headaches are associated with skin abnormalities. An example is that some people with neurofibromatosis, which is associated with particular types of birthmarks, are prone to develop certain kinds of brain tumors. Your doctor should ask you about birthmarks: Are there dark patches on your child's skin? Light patches that never tan? Unusual bumps? Show the doctor these areas.

Heart, lungs and abdomen. These should be examined in the way you are familiar with from other visits to the doctor. Sometimes headaches can happen because of illness in other parts of the body, and so your doctor will need to examine these areas.

The head itself. Physically touching the child's head and neck area, obvious as it may seem, may be forgotten in the rush to test how the brain is actually functioning. However, there are several important features of this part of the examination. Infections and bleeding inside the head can cause a stiff neck, so having the child touch his chin to his chest is a way to demonstrate whether her neck is stiff. Your doctor should also feel whether your child's neck muscles themselves are tense—sometimes tight neck muscles put tension on the scalp, where pain receptors lie (see the discussion on tension headaches in Chapter 2). Although the condition is rare, the occipital nerves, which come up around the base of the skull, can get inflamed, causing severe headaches. Touching the areas where these nerves lie can reproduce the headache, and therefore make the diagnosis.

• • •

Now, we turn to actually examining the functioning of the brain.

Eyes. The saying goes, "The eyes are the window of the soul." That may be, but neurologists are just as happy to use them to look into your brain. Eyes are directly connected to the brain. As a matter of fact, the only nerve that can actually be seen is the optic nerve, which connects the eyes to the brain. Doctors can see this nerve by shining a thin beam of light into a patient's eye with a tool called an ophthalmoscope.

Your child's visual acuity may be tested. Poor vision is one cause of headaches (see the discussion on eyestrain headaches in Chapter 2). This is done using the eye chart that is probably familiar to everyone. Of course, younger children will not be able to cooperate with this test.

Visual fields will be tested as well as possible given your child's age. Your visual field is what you can see, both in front of you and to the sides. We can all see a particular amount before we have to turn our heads, and that is our visual field. Testing visual fields is important because so much of the brain is devoted to analyzing vision. So, if there is a problem involving part of the brain, there is a good chance that it will affect the visual fields. Your doctor can test visual fields several different ways, but the usual way to do it is to have your child look straight at the doctor's nose while the doctor waves different objects on each side to see if your child can see them. With an older child, the doctor might ask the child to tell how many fingers are being held up. But as you can imagine, it would be impossible to test a baby this way! The best you can do with a baby is to try to focus his attention on some object (a toy or a face) and then wave another toy in a different part of his visual field, seeing if you can distract him. If you can, then you assume he sees in that part of his visual field.

The doctor will also examine your child's eyes themselves. The pupillary reflex—seeing how pupils react to light—is probably something everyone has experienced during an exam. Testing this reflex can give important information; the pathways involved are sometimes affected by tumors. Your doctor will try to look in the back of your child's eye with an ophthalmoscope. The doctor is actually trying to see the optic nerve—the nerve that connects the eyeball to the brain—where it comes out in the back of the eyeball. Since there is a direct connection to the brain there, an increase in pressure inside your child's head (sometimes from tumors or other masses, sometimes from excess fluid inside the brain) can cause changes in the optic nerve. Sometimes, however, the changes caused by the increased pressure are slow to appear. If the headache has been going on for a short time (a couple of weeks or less, usually) the eyes might look normal.

The way the eyes move is also important. Your doctor will have your child move his eyes in all directions. Then the doctor will look to see that the eyes are not restricted in any way, and that they are moving in synchrony. Again, tumors or increased pressure can sometimes cause restricted movement. If the restriction in movement is greater in one eye, double vision can result. Your child may not see precisely two images but may have the sensation of blurry vision. Blurry vision can result from other reasons, however, and its presence is not necessarily a cause for alarm.

Other nerves of the head. The cranial nerves conduct impulses from your brain to your face. Besides your eyes, they control nose and mouth function as well as facial sensation and movements, so all these functions should be tested. Your child may be asked to identify a scent such as peppermint. An inability to smell most often indicates a stuffy nose, but this can also give information about brain damage after an accident (injuries can occur to the nerve fibers involved in smell) as well as about possible tumors located in the area between the nose and the brain. Your doctor may ask whether your child feels sensation on his face, or may ask him to move his face in a particular way to demonstrate the strength of the facial muscles (or, he may just collect this information by observing your child).

Reflexes. Next comes a fairly fun part of the exam—reflexes! Everybody likes to see their legs jump when the doctor taps their knees, but few people really understand what it's all about. The reflexes are composed of an input and an output. The input comes when the reflex hammer taps your knee. Receptors sense a stretch and transmit that information to the spinal cord, which in turn sends an output signal to your muscle to contract and relieve the tension on the stretch receptor. Reflexes like this aren't just present at your knees. There are reflexes in your arms and at your ankles as well. All operate on the same principle.

What does this have to do with the brain and headaches? The brain actually modulates this reflex—it dampens it. So, if part of your child's brain is injured or compressed by a tumor, your doctor can detect it on exam by looking for a change in reflexes. For example, a problem on the left side of the brain might cause extra-bouncy reflexes on the right side of the body (remember, the left side of the brain controls the right side of the body and vice versa).

Motor skills. Another fun part of the exam is the motor skills part of the exam. Here your child should get the chance to show the doctor how strong he is. The doctor will test strength by asking the child to resist pressure on different muscle groups. For example, your child may be asked to flex his arms while the doctor tries to extend them. For younger children who cannot follow directions well, this test is mainly done by observation. Does the child seem to use both sides of his body equally while crawling or climbing? Again, as strength is partly controlled by the brain, testing it will help show whether there are problems in the brain. The doctor will also try to get a sense of the tone of the muscles by seeing how flexible your child's arms and legs are.

Sensory. Brains also interpret sensations, and these sensations must be tested as well. This is very difficult to test in babies and young children. However, older children will be able to identify (with their eyes closed) a coin placed in their hands. Another common test checks for the ability to recognize vibrations at the toes. Finally, the doctor may move your child's big toe up or down (again, with the child's eyes closed), and ask which way the toe is moving. The ability to distinguish where body parts are in space without visual cues is called proprioception. All these different tests of sensation check different types of pathways in the brain.

Coordination. Finally, tests of coordination should be done. Coordination is controlled by the back part of the brain, an area called the cerebellum. This area is frequently involved in tumors in children, so it is important to test. The doctor will try to entice children to grab or touch something, and will look to see if this is done in a reasonably coordinated fashion. Of course, the ability to reach out and grab improves with age; babies don't even start to be able to do so before a few months of age, and at that point they are rarely successful. Babies are naturally uncoordinated! But by about six months of age, grabbing should be much easier. A six-month-old can usually transfer an object from hand to hand, and it just keeps getting better from then on. The doctor can look to see whether each side is equally coordinated and whether either side has less coordinated movements than should be expected for age. By the time your child is two he should definitely be able to smoothly point to a small target. If your child is old enough, he will probably be asked to do the finger-nose-finger test, in which he points to his own nose, then to the doctor's finger, then to his nose again, as fast as possible. This is a very good test of coordination. Another test that is often done is to see whether your child can perform rapid alternating movements smoothly, such as tapping his fingers together rhythmically. This is another cerebellar function.

• • •

These are some of the basic tests that can be done. Your child may have most of these tests done or your doctor may decide to do fewer tests. There may be additional tests done that are not described here. The general rule is that the older the child, the more detailed the tests that can be done, because your child will be better able to cooperate. The younger the child, the more you may have to rely on other tests such as CT scans or MRIs, because the physical exam is not as reliable.

THE DIAGNOSIS

How does a doctor go about making a diagnosis of what is causing a headache? Every doctor has his own method of thinking about the *differential diagnosis*—the list of all the possible causes of the headache—and coming up with what he thinks best fits the situation. Here is a basic framework:

One major decision your doctor has to make is: are these headaches emergencies? Will the child suffer serious injury or die if his headaches are not diagnosed and treated right now? Or can these headaches be diagnosed and treated over the next few days, weeks, or months?

How does the doctor figure out whether the headache is an emergency?

One factor that is helpful in making a diagnosis is the *time* over which the patient has suffered from the headaches. Severe headaches that have been present for only hours or days may be emergencies. Headache emergencies include bleeding in the head (for example, from aneurysms) and infections in the head (meningitis or encephalitis). Both of these conditions cause a stiff neck, making it hard for a patient to move his head forward toward his chest. Both conditions can also cause people to have altered consciousness, becoming sleepy or even comatose. So any headache that has a new onset and involves those features is an emergency, requiring treatment in the emergency room of a hospital.

However, most people who come to an office for headaches have a more chronic headache problem. They have usually been suffering from the headaches for weeks, months, or years. As a general rule, if your child has an actively bleeding aneurysm or meningitis, the time course of the headache will be short rather than long, so the longer the headache goes on the less of an emergency it's going to be.

Let's think about headaches that have been ongoing, without a break, for days or weeks. The next most important factor to think about is the severity of the pain: Is it getting worse? That could represent something growing in the head like a tumor. The doctor would also look not only for physical causes such as a mass in the brain or an enlarging vascular malformation, but he would also consider whether social or psychological issues could be playing a role.

What if the headache has been off and on for days or weeks but generally is not getting much worse? This is the most frequent pattern of headaches seen in an office setting. If the headache fits this category, the next thing to consider is the pattern of the headache—when it comes and when it goes. Headaches that come and go, especially if they have been around for years, are usually "safer" headaches, those that can be treated more slowly or on a "watch and wait" basis. There are exceptions to this, however. If a recurrent headache is associated with certain body positions, such as lying down, this is cause for concern. A positional component is associated with headaches from colloid cysts (see Chapter 2), which are rare but could be fatal. Another concerning pattern is headaches in association with exercise, which could indicate vascular problems (although this pattern can also be associated with more benign problems).

If the headaches are not getting worse, are they getting better? That probably means that you could wait, not do any studies now, and see if the headaches recur.

Migraines, the most frequent headaches seen in the office, can fit any of the above patterns, so how will the decision be made to either try treatment with migraine medications or attempt further tests (like a scan)? Your doctor will probably think about what a "perfect" story for migraines is, one that fits every single feature most commonly seen in migraines. To briefly review Chapter 3, these factors include: strong family history for migraines, seeing little shimmering lights around the time the headache starts, throwing up, and having one-sided throbbing headaches that shift sides. If your child's headache is absolutely classic for migraines, and a normal neurologic exam rules out other problems (such as a tumor), the doctor may not do any further testing and may treat your child for migraines. However, especially in children, most migraine stories are not "perfect" at all. Every doctor has to decide individually how far away from the standard migraine history one can get and still make a correct diagnosis.

Your doctor will need to think about symptoms that may be associated with the headache as well. As stated above, a stiff neck might propel the headache into emergency status, but other worrisome features include throwing up or seizures. Both of these features are fairly common with brain tumors, although kids who throw up with headaches are statistically much more likely to have migraines. There may be other unrelated medical conditions that can cause your child to have a headache.

Since migraines are common and often run in families, family history will be considered. If the headaches could be migraines based on the symptoms, and if there is a strong family history of migraine, that could help make the diagnosis and alleviate the need for imaging studies.

So far, we have used only the historical information to make decisions. What about the physical examination? How does the doctor fit in that information?

Most often, the exam will be entirely normal. If there are no concerning features of the headaches and the exam is normal, there is almost no reason to proceed with more testing. In contrast, if there are any problems on the exam, even if the history is not so bad, there is almost every reason to do further testing to explain it. Restrictions in the visual fields or swelling of the optic nerves, for example, could indicate a problem such as high cerebrospinal fluid pressure or a slowly growing tumor, even though the headaches themselves from the tumor may not have been so bad.

So to summarize, doctors go through the different factors on the history and combine that with the findings on the physical exam. They will try to sort out what is an emergency and what is not. They will then make a presumptive diagnosis, and will either confirm it with tests if appropriate (see below) or treat the patient based on their working diagnosis. Hopefully they will then see the patient improve, which will confirm the diagnosis! If not, then the doctor has to think again.

CONFIRMATORY TESTING

The doctor has gathered his information. He has taken the history—what you and your child have said about the headaches—and done a physical exam, looking for clues as to why your child might have headaches. Now comes the moment of truth: Does he know with reasonable certainty what is causing your child's headaches? Or does he need to do more testing to find out?

Let's turn to the phrase "reasonable certainty." A doctor does not always know with 100 percent certainty what the problem is. This is especially true in neurology, where the clinical symptom (the headache) can't be seen and the brain can be examined only by deduction. As discussed in Chapters 2 and 3, defining where the different headache syndromes begin and end is hard, too, because the syndromes are not well defined in children.

Even the very best doctors and top specialists can't always say what is causing a case of headaches. Doctors use the information they find out from the history and physical exam, combine it with their reasoning and experience, and then do their best to come up with a diagnosis.

It would be easy if, after taking in all the information, the doctor could make a presumptive diagnosis—migraine, for example—and then get a quick blood test to make sure. This would be like checking the answer in an answer book. But in reality there is no answer book. With the exception of certain very specific problems that can be seen on a CT or MRI scan (tumors, aneurysms, and the like), there is no objective answer. In most cases what you receive is an opinion about whether your child is suffering from migraines or tension headaches. As technologies improve this may change, but this is the current state of medical knowledge.

On the other hand, you want to know *with certainty* what is causing your child's headaches. How do you resolve this conflict?

The closest thing doctors have to an answer book is time. Over time, new symptoms might develop which will better explain the symptoms. For example, a child might start out with fairly nonspecific headaches and then develop headaches associated with seeing little flashing lights, a symptom almost always associated with migraines. Or a physical examination could subsequently reveal additional symptoms, such as weakness in the limbs, that would offer more information.

But as a parent, this wait-and-see approach can sometimes be cause for alarm. Is it OK to wait? What if there is an aneurysm causing the headaches? What if there is a tumor? How does a doctor decide whether it's OK to wait?

This is where trust in the doctor and his experience comes in.

But how do you know if your doctor is trustworthy? Figuring out who to trust is probably the hardest issue to deal with as a patient. It is especially hard to trust in a nebulous field like neurology and headaches, where there is a lack of clear objective data that you can see.

Should you trust your doctor

Here are some questions to ask yourself:

- Did the doctor spend enough time with you so you felt like you discussed the problem fully?
- Did you feel that he was on "automatic pilot," or did he ask you questions geared to your particular situation?
- Was the exam perfunctory or detailed?
- Did the doctor take time to explain why he thought his diagnosis was right?
- Did the doctor's assessment agree with your own gut feelings about the headaches?

Once you have chosen a doctor and gone to see him, you will then still have to decide whether to trust his assessment. Hopefully this book will help you do so, but to some degree you will still have to trust your intuition.

The answer often is tied into how you choose a doctor in the first place. You might have picked a doctor based on his reputation. He might be nationally or locally famous for figuring out headaches. But what if he's having an "off day"? What if he sees so many patients that you feel rushed, and you're concerned that he didn't really understand the problem fully? What if you find out he spends 98 percent of his time doing research on the subject rather than seeing patients?

More than likely in this age of insurance controls, you didn't have much of a choice in who you went to see. You saw your primary care doctor, or perhaps your doctor referred you to a specialist. But how much trust can you put in a referral? Nowadays, many primary care doctors don't have much choice in who *they* refer you to either, especially if they are part of a closed health plan (like an HMO). Even if there is a choice, how do you know that your doctor didn't pick your specialist based on who he likes to eat lunch with?

You might be asking: Why not just do a CT or MRI scan on everybody? That way, no tumor or other problem will be missed, and I won't have to worry about whether my child's doctor is a good one or not.

There are many reasons why these scans cannot be done on every patient with a headache, even on every child with a headache. One easy answer: Society cannot afford to do this. Headaches are so common that it would be impossible to scan everybody. Insurance companies would go broke (or not cover headaches). New scanners would have to be built, for there would be no way the current amount could accommodate everyone (or, you'd have to wait months or years to get a scan). And because the scans themselves can be uncomfortable and frightening, especially for children, patients would suffer needlessly. Incidental findings unrelated to the cause of the headaches would be found, often leading to further testing and worry for the patient (and if undiscovered, the vast majority of these findings would never cause any problems anyway). And for what? Physicians generally have an excellent rate of accurate diagnoses without the tests. In addition, the tests will not help distinguish certain types of headaches: For example, both migraine headaches and tension headaches cause no significant abnormalities on MRI scans.

Even with screening by a physician, most tests ordered will be normal. Although insurance companies probably aren't happy about the number of tests ordered, physicians do not only obtain tests that they think will show a problem. They would miss many abnormalities that way. They obtain tests on anybody who might possibly have a problem based on the history and physical. The vast majority of tests that they order show normal findings.

Many physicians will order a scan if:

- The neurologic exam is abnormal.
- There might be bleeding or infection.
- There might be a tumor or other mass in the head.
- There is a strong family history of aneurysms or other vascular malformations.
- The headaches are not suggestive of a benign process.
- Your child has been treated without success and he is getting worse.
- The headaches are significantly changing and/or worsening.

• • •

Let's talk about these tests in further detail.

CT scans. CT scans are cross-sectional X rays taken of the brain. They are pronounced "C.T." scan or "CAT" scan; a CAT scan is the same thing as a CT scan. CT stands for "computed tomography." The patient lies down, with her head placed in the center of a plastic-and-metal circle called the scanner. The scanner makes whirring and clanking noises as it takes the "pictures," while the patient has to lie still. Just as with a regular camera, if the subject of the picture moves the images will come out blurry. The whole process should take less than fifteen minutes.

X rays are sent through the head, every 5 mm, from the bottom of the brain to the top (or every 10 mm, from the top to the bottom—whatever parameters the technician sets). The tissues within and around the brain absorb the X rays in different amounts. The machine will record this as black-and-white shades. For example, blood and bone tissues look white, air and cerebrospinal fluid (CSF) looks black, and the brain itself is represented by different shades of gray. Sometimes a special dye will be used to help certain problems stand out. This dye is iodine based. Many people who are allergic to shellfish are also allergic to iodine, so if your child has a history of shellfish allergies, let your doctor or the CT technologist know *before* a "with-contrast" study is done. The pictures will be recorded, printed out on special film, and sent to a radiologist (a specialist in looking at and interpreting pictures of the body). Your child's doctor will either receive a report from the radiologist or, ideally, will also get to look at the scans himself (see Figure 6, a picture of a CT scan).

Because CT scans are relatively quicker than MRI scans, they are used in emergency situations. CT scans are very good at showing bleeding, and can also be used to tell if a mass is deforming the brain or if hydrocephalus (too much water on the inside of the brain; see Chapter 2) is developing. The downside is that they are not as good as MRI scans at showing problems in the cerebellum or brainstem, where tumors often form in young children (the skull bones make those areas harder to see). Generally, CT scans give a much less detailed picture of the various parts of the brain than MRI scans.

Depending on what the doctor suspects, CT scans can still be very useful in the evaluation of headache. Because they are so quick, CT scans are particularly useful for young children who cannot sit still (an MRI will require sedation for those cannot remain still for an hour or so). Sometimes a CT will be chosen over an MRI just because of this factor. Although a CT scan can show whether hydrocephalus is taking place because of a tumor, it may miss small tumors themselves. The radiation dose of a scan is another factor to consider (in comparison, MRI scans do not

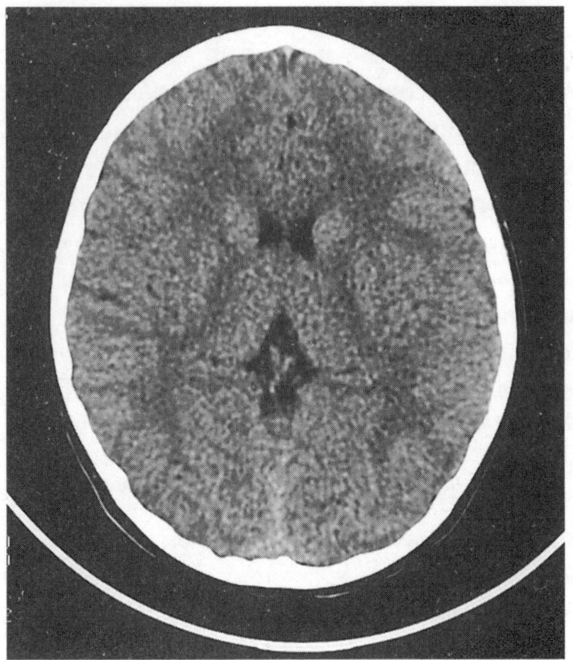

Figure 6. A CT scan.

use X rays) but as the dose is small, this should not really be a significant factor in your decision.

MRI scans. MRI (Magnetic Resonance Imaging) scans use a different type of technology. The machine creates strong magnetic pulses, which energize the hydrogen nuclei in the brain. The machine then uses radio waves to help read where the various amounts of hydrogen atoms are present. Hydrogen atoms are found in all biological tissues and water, and the different amounts of hydrogen in different parts of the brain and cerebrospinal fluid will cause differences in the radio waves. This information can then be translated by the machine into pictures. Like the CT scan, these are printed out on special film and first read by a radiologist. Also as in CT scans, sometimes a special dye will be given that can highlight certain abnormalities. This dye is not iodine based, but it can sometimes interact adversely with certain medications for diabetes.

MRIs will sometimes have an MRA (Magnetic Resonance Angiogram) added on. You can think of this as an MRI that is especially tuned to blood vessels, because the machine looks for flow in the arteries of the head. An MRV (Magnetic Resonance Venogram) is another variation, which looks for problems especially in the veins of the head.

Look at the picture of an MRI scan (Figure 7) and compare it to the CT scan (Figure 6). As you can see, the MRI scan is much more detailed than a CT scan. However, there are some things that are easier to read on a CT scan. Bones, as well as blood, are seen very well on a CT scan. These are less visible on MRI scans (although MRI scans can provide better images for bleeding that has been present for more than a day or so).

MRIs are superior to CT scans in many ways. They are generally the imaging study of choice to look for problems such as tumors in the tissues of the brain. They are especially good at looking for small tumors that might not deform the brain much (however, these small tumors are less likely to cause headaches, more likely to cause seizures).

However, a major drawback of MRIs is that they take a long time to do—at least an hour or more—and the child has to be still during this time. Young children or uncooperative children often require sedation to get through it. The child's entire body has to be slid into the scanner, rather than having a machine just around his head. This results in not much of the child being visible. Sometimes the combination of sedation plus not being able to closely observe the child can be dangerous—a child could stop breathing, or throw up and choke on the vomit in the scanner without anybody knowing. If possible, try to have the scan done in a center that has a lot of experience with sedating children if your child will require sedation.

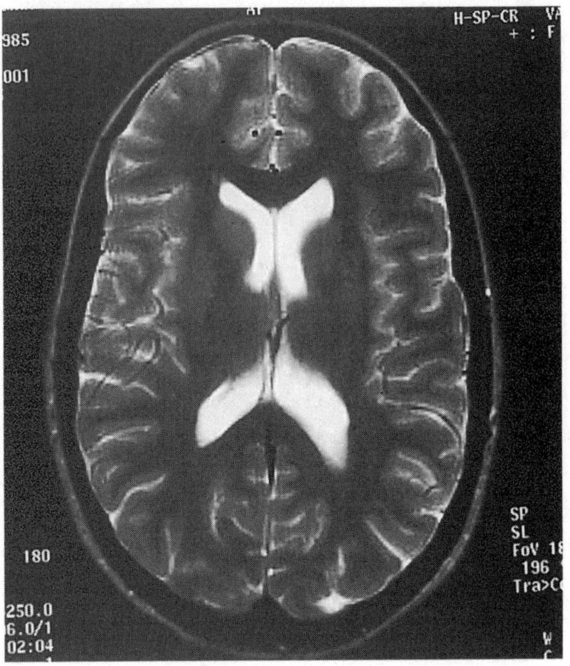

Figure 7. A MRI scan.

Finally, there is the cost issue. MRIs are more expensive than CT scans; an MRI can cost more than a thousand dollars as compared to a few hundred for a CT scan. For families who are paying out of pocket, this could be important. Of course every parent wants the best for his or her children, but sometimes a CT scan will do just as well. If cost is an issue for your family, be sure to discuss this with your doctor.

What about other tests, other than taking pictures of the brain? Blood tests are usually not very helpful in determining the cause of the headache. In certain situations, though, they can be revealing. Headaches caused by general medical problems are usually diagnosed by blood tests. For example, if a patient is anemic, she might have headaches (in addition to being unusually tired). A complete blood count (CBC) would show a low amount of red blood cells, which would usually be treated by iron replacement. Low thyroid function may also cause headaches. Certain types of infections that are associated with headaches can also be diagnosed with the aid of blood tests.

Lumbar puncture. There is yet another test used to diagnose headaches called a lumbar puncture (LP) or spinal tap (often abbreviated to "tap"). In certain situations, this is the only test that can show the cause of the problem. On the downside, it involves a needle in the back. Most kids—and most adults—given the choice, would rather not go through it. Luckily, diagnosis of most headaches does not require a lumbar puncture.

The test looks at the cerebrospinal fluid (CSF) that bathes the brain and spinal cord. CSF is produced by specialized cells in the middle of the brain. The fluid flows out of the brain through several channels and then circulates around the outside of the brain, between the brain and the lining on the inside of the skull. This space is contiguous with the space between the outside of the spinal cord and the vertebrae. It is much easier and much less dangerous to sample the fluid from someone's back than from someone's head, and so the back is where the fluid is accessed. There is a space in the lower back where this is accomplished without hitting the spinal cord itself (which actually ends closer to the middle of the back).

The child may or may not be sedated. Very young children who cannot cooperate will require sedation, but older cooperative children will be able to get through the test without sedation. The child will be placed on his side, curled up in the fetal position. The object of this position is to curl the spine enough so that the spaces between the vertebrae will be easy to feel. The doctor will clean off the area with an iodine compound, then will place a needle between the lower lumbar vertebrae, with the tip of the needle landing a few centimeters below where the spinal cord ends. The fluid will come out of the needle. The opening pressure, which is the pressure of the very first few drops of fluid as it comes out, is important to determine and is obtained with a tool attached to the doctor's end of the needle. The fluid is then collected into sterile tubes and sent to the lab for testing.

If all goes well, this test is absolutely bloodless. Inserting the needle can usually be done without blood, and the fluid obtained is normally as clear as water. However, you may see blood if the needle has to be repositioned or if, on the way to its target, it hits a blood vessel (the blood vessels in this area are small and puncturing them does not cause damage). Junior medical residents are often rewarded with a bottle of champagne if they do a tap with a red blood cell count of zero! (Nobody gets red wine for a tap with a high red cell count.)

How can I help my child get through a lumbar puncture?

- Tell the doctor ahead of time if your child has a known allergy to iodine. An iodine-like compound is usually used to sterilize the patient's back in the beginning of the procedure.
- Remain calm. If you show your fears, your child will respond accordingly and become fearful himself.
- Some doctors let parents watch the procedure; others are uncomfortable with this. If you are allowed to watch, hold your child's hand and talk to him about comfortable and familiar things that will make him relax and even smile.
- Ask the doctor to give you and your child a "play by play," telling you what is going to happen during the procedure. The child is facing away from the doctor and can't see what is going on; likewise, if you are in the room you will be positioned so you will best comfort your child and may not have the best view of what the doctor is doing. You will both feel more comfortable hearing the doctor explain what is happening.

- If you see blood or if or if there is another complication, remain calm and do not draw the child's attention to it.
- If you know you have a tendency to faint in stressful situations or if you know you faint at the side of blood, do not plan on being in the room during the procedure. Having a parent faint is stressful for everyone!

The pressure of the fluid and the content of it both yield important information. Why would knowing the pressure of the fluid be of use? A condition called pseudotumor cerebri (also known as benign intracranial hypertension) causes headaches because the pressure of the fluid inside the head is too high. Nobody knows exactly why this is the case, but it seems to involve an overproduction of fluid. Normally, CSF is constantly being produced and reabsorbed at an even rate. If there is an overproduction, however, the reabsorption cells can't keep up, and pressure builds up. So the opening pressure measured during the test will be high—sometimes very high. Normally CSF pressure is under 200 mm H_20, but in some cases of pseudotumor the fluid will be 500 mm H_20 or higher. Doing the tap and taking off some of the fluid makes people who have this condition feel better, because it relieves the pressure. If their headaches come back they may actually ask for more spinal taps! Usually, though, this condition is relieved with medication rather than repeated taps. It is an important condition to treat, because if untreated the elevated pressure will lead to problems with vision (see Chapter 2 for more details). Pseudotumor is not too rare (most neurologists will see several cases during their career), but a related and very rare cause of headaches stems from low CSF pressure (thought to occur mainly in adults).

What about the content of the fluid? The content of the fluid is analyzed in a laboratory. There are many tests that could be run, but standard ones usually include protein and sugar (glucose) content. In addition, microbiological tests looking for inflamed cells are run. The red blood cell count of the fluid is also noted. If the red blood cell count is high, that either means blood caused by the procedure got mixed in with the sample or that there was bleeding in the head before the procedure started.

Specialized laboratory tests can determine if the high red blood cell count is from the actual puncture and not the child's condition.

• • •

This chapter should have given you a little more information about what might go on in the doctor's office. You can use this information to prepare your child for what may happen, as well as to make better use of the time you spend with the doctor. These facts will help you give the doctor appropriate information about your child's headaches, understand the examination a little better, and then be able to talk to the doctor about his diagnosis.

CHAPTER 7

The Intractable Headache

The Unwanted Family Member

Sometimes, despite everyone's best efforts, some children have headaches that are very difficult to control. The headaches may occur with great frequency or severity, or they may develop into a single headache that never seems to go away, no matter what you do. Long-lasting headaches are called *migraine status* or *chronic daily headache.*

Such headaches are very difficult, not just on the child who is experiencing them but on the entire family. Many emotions come into play, especially at the beginning of the headache. The following are some examples that may strike a chord with you, voices I've heard from parents, siblings, and grandparents.

WORRY

- Is there something dangerously wrong with my child?
- Is my brother/sister going to die?
- Is my doctor doing the right things for my child, or should I seek a second opinion or a more expert opinion?
- I'm losing so much time at work and so much money staying home with my child, what are we going to do?
- Should I be demanding more tests for my child?
- Is my daughter/son doing the right thing for my grandchild?
- Maybe he really has a brain tumor.

GUILT

- Maybe something I'm doing is causing this.
- Maybe something I should have done could have avoided this.
- Maybe if I hadn't gotten into a fight with my brother/sister he wouldn't be so sick right now.
- Maybe if I hadn't disciplined him he would be feeling fine right now.
- Maybe if I had just stayed at home with him that first day, this wouldn't have happened.
- If I hadn't let him drink that soda, this probably wouldn't have happened.
- I thought he was just whining in the beginning.
- How can I worry about money I'm missing from not going to work, when my child is so sick?
- This is my fault for trying to hold a job and raise a child at the same time.
- I'm tired of taking care of him; I must be a bad mother/father.
- Why couldn't this be happening to me instead of him?
- It's my fault, since I have migraines and I passed on the migraine genes to him.
- I'm not devoting enough energy to my spouse or other children during this time.

ANGER/BLAME

- If he would just get his act together...
- If he would just not be such a wimp...
- He's dragging this on just to irritate me.
- My husband/wife just doesn't understand what he's going through.
- My husband/wife just doesn't understand what I'm going through with the child.

- My husband/wife is angry at me for letting things get to this point.
- My husband/wife is angry at me for being too hard/easy on the child.
- My brother/sister would be fine if he would just wake up and get to school.
- My brother/sister is scaring my parents and that makes me angry.
- My brother/sister is scaring me and that makes me angry.
- My parents don't even notice me any more; they just think about my brother/sister's headaches.
- I'm going to lose my job because of this kid's headaches.
- Everyone thinks I'm being a bad parent.
- Everyone thinks I'm too much of a worrier.
- It's the teacher's fault: She didn't let my child take his medication, and now she's angry at me for not bringing him to school when he's in pain.
- Mom is missing my school play so she can stay home and take care of my brother.
- My grandchild would be fine if his father/mother would take better care of him.

SUSPICION

- He's not really in pain.
- He's lazy.
- He's just doing this to get out of school/chores.
- He's just doing this for more attention.
- He's fine, without a headache, when it's time to do something he wants. When it's something I want to do, his headache somehow always gets in the way.

FRUSTRATION AND HELPLESSNESS.

- When will this end?
- Why won't anything fix this headache?
- What can I do to make this be over?
- Why is he not even getting better?
- This is never going to end.
- How the heck am I going to ever get to work?
- The doctors don't know anything.
- All the medicines just make him feel worse, and we are never going to find anything that works.
- Just when I think he's getting better, he gets worse again.
- There's nothing I can do.

EXHAUSTION

- I'm working extra hours so my wife can stay home and take care of our son.
- I'm doing extra work around the house so my husband can spend time with our child.
- I'm still trying to be a normal mom for my other children.
- This is really hard on all of us.

If you have a child with intractable headaches, your family has experienced a lot of these emotions and thoughts, and probably more. None of these emotions are positive ones; they are all very stressful and difficult for families to cope with. Sometimes, people will experience a lot of these emotions at once, even though they seem to be contradictory. For example, a working mother (who may already have feelings of guilt for leaving her child) may simultaneously experience worry about how the doctors' bills will be paid, anger at the child for not feeling better, guilt at worrying over money when her child is sick, and frustration that he's not getting better. Dad may feel tired of taking care of the child, anger that he's not getting better, mad at the doctors for not doing enough, and frustrated with Mom for "babying" the child too much.

If Mom gets stressed out by her child's headaches, what then happens to her relationship with Dad? While it's possible that Mom and Dad may pull together as a team in situations like this, often Mom and Dad will get upset with each other (consciously or subconsciously). For example, Dad may resent losing some of the attention that Mom had previously given him. The stress of a chronic illness in the house may bring to the surface any previously simmering tensions. Both parents may take this opportunity to blame the headache on the other's parenting "deficiencies." Dad may have had previous thoughts that Mom tended to be too easy on the child, and the headaches will reinforce those thoughts: *My wife has created a weak child, and that's why he has headaches.* Mom may feel that Dad has been too distant or too hard on the child, and may believe that the headaches are a result of this behavior: *My child has headaches to get his father's attention.*

And where does this leave other children in the family, those who are not suffering from headaches? Mom and Dad's attentions are now focused on their sibling, and Mom and Dad are tense with each other. *Mom and Dad are exhausted, cranky, and snapping at each other and at me!* It is very easy for other children in the family to feel alone and left out at a time when they, too, are experiencing complicated emotions. They are worried about their affected sibling, but they may be angry with him at the same time. Household tasks that their brother or sister was expected to do may now fall to them, and they may feel resentful. They see their brother or sister being waited on and catered to, while they still have to go to school and do all the work. They may view their ill sibling as being the cause of all these problems, and they experience the very difficult-to-process emotions of being angry at someone you also love and are worried about.

Parents and siblings are also angry at the general disruption of their family life. The headache can become a very intrusive presence, having more power than anything else in the family to influence decision making. Here are some examples from daily life:

- We can't go to the park because it might make the headache worse.
- We can't go to the party because he has a headache.
- I can't go to your soccer game because I have to take your brother to the doctor for the headache.
- Please empty the trash. I know it's not your job, but your sister has a headache.
- Please be quiet! You're making your sister's headache worse!
- He can't go to school yet. The headache might come back.
- We can't buy that. I've missed so much work because of that headache.
- Maybe I should just quit my job and stay home permanently if these headaches are going to continue to be a problem.

The child experiencing these headaches is experiencing mixed emotions of his own. He has the pain to deal with, of course, but he also has to deal with the family members around him. He, too, is feeling worried: *What's wrong with me?* Guilt: *It's my fault I have this headache and am causing all these problems.* Anger/blame: *Why does this have to happen to me?* Suspicion: *Maybe if I tried harder I could end this.* Frustration/helplessness: *I'm never going to get better.* Exhaustion: *I just want to get back to my normal routine.*

He is also experiencing a further emotion: loneliness. *Nobody understands what I'm going through. I never see my friends anymore.*

Throughout the process, your child and your family will be interacting with community members; not just medical personnel, but teachers, family friends, coaches, and others. The more disrupted your family life becomes because of the headache problem, the more the family will feel isolated from their usual routines and relationships with these other community members. Decisions may have to be made that would have been unthinkable prior to the headache onset, most notably with school. For example, parents of a student previously getting all "A's" may have to meet with the school to decide what to do, as the student is now failing because of absenteeism, failure to turn in homework assignments, and poor concentration. Should the "A" student have to repeat the year because of these headaches?

And what happens to your child and family as you journey through the medical process? Your child may have to undergo a number of tests (MRI scans, lumbar puncture, and more) that may be frightening and painful. He may be placed on a series of medications with bad side effects. Your child may run the risk of overtesting: The more medical tests that are run, the more likely one is to turn out abnormal, generating more tests (even though they may turn out to be irrelevant). You may miss work because of doctor's appointments, not to mention staying home with a sick child. Your family may experience financial hardships, not just because of missed work but because of costs of medication, tests, and specialist visits.

Here is the case of Erica, a girl with a highly intractable migraine, and some of the problems that she and her family experienced. This is an example of an extremely long course of headache with a lot of complicating factors, but many of the issues are present in less remarkable cases.

• • •

Erica was thirteen years old when she first came to the attention of a neurologist. She had a history of migraine headaches off and on since she was about seven years old. Her mother, too, had a history of migraine headaches, and her father had a history of cluster headaches. However, until recently Erica had done quite well. She was a superb student, described as athletic and outgoing, and she was on several sports teams. Medically, she was quite healthy. A couple of years earlier there had been some concern that Erica was anorexic; she seemed to be strongly focused on maintaining her weight below a certain point. However, that had seemed to get better with dietary counseling and removal of the scales from the home. She lived at home with both parents and two younger siblings. Nothing out of the ordinary had been going on at home, no particular stressors on the family were known.

Erica's headaches used to only occur in the fall, but this year they had begun in the summer and seemed to be more intense. She was brought to her primary care physician every week or so, and multiple medications were tried with no effect. Within two months, three CT scans were done. These were followed by a lumbar puncture. Between the headaches, the medical visits, and the testing, she had already missed significant amounts of school by October, and her mom decided to home-school her. This caused a financial hardship to the family, but they saw no other options.

By November, she was admitted to a hospital four hours' drive from the family home. Mom stayed at the hospital with Erica, and Dad became the primary caretaker to the other children, while still maintaining his full-time work schedule. At the hospital Erica was tried on some intravenous medications, which seemed to stop her headache. The neurologists taking care of her could find no other reasons why Erica was having headaches and felt that she was in the middle of a bad migraine. A psychiatrist was consulted, who felt that Erica would probably benefit from stress management counseling. Erica was discharged after about a week and was headache-free when she was discharged. However, within two days of being home her headaches returned in full force.

At home she grew more and more inconsolable. She stayed home in a dark room most of the time. She didn't see any of her friends. At first she would talk to them on the phone but then felt that that was "too much." She cried a lot, and she did not want to shower or even change her clothes. Erica was unable to do any schoolwork or exercise; it worsened her headache. She felt incapable of doing anything. Her grandmother came to live with the family to help out. Erica even had her mercury dental fillings extracted, but there was still no change in her condition.

More medications were tried. Erica was by now on a combination of medications, all of which had side effects. One particularly difficult day, when she was in a lot of pain and had taken a lot of medications, she had a seizure. She was walking through a doorway, collapsed, hit her head on the ground, stiffened, and convulsed. That generated a series of additional tests. She had an EEG, which was done to look for an area of her brain that might be generating seizures. It was abnormal. However, since it was only one seizure and since some of the medications that she was on for her headaches had the side effect of causing seizures in some people, her doctors elected not to place her on antiseizure medication. She had a MRI scan of her brain. A minor abnormality was seen, but it was not thought to explain her headaches.

By mid-January, Erica began to have problems with repeated vomiting. By mid-March, she could not keep anything down, and was rehospitalized to treat dehydration and try again to control her headaches. Gastroenterologists were consulted to make sure that nothing was wrong with Erica's digestive tract. They did a number of tests and found a small ulcer in Erica's stomach that may have been due to the medications she was taking. Erica was placed on additional medications to treat the ulcer. Specialists in pain were consulted, and they thought that Erica may have developed an addiction to some of her headache medications and may also be suffering rebound headaches from the medications. Headache medications were switched. Erica did not improve. However, the medical personnel she came in contact with noticed that Erica was exhibiting some strange behavior—she would be crying in seeming agony from the pain, then stop immediately when somebody entered the room and started talking to her. Finally, pain medications were cancelled altogether, except for acetaminophen. Erica did not seem any worse. Psychiatrists were re-consulted to assess whether some of Erica's pain and pain behaviors stemmed from stress or anxiety.

The psychiatrists noted that Erica was throwing up constantly and not eating. They began to consider that Erica's current behavior may have been influenced by her past history of anorexia. She was admitted to the inpatient psychiatry ward essentially as an anorexia patient, despite the misgivings of her mother and herself, but both agreed to give it a try.

On the ward, Erica was encouraged and expected to go to the school that was held there. She was given responsibilities. She was rewarded when she did not spend time focusing on her pain. She was given relaxation and imagery exercises to do and was encouraged to exercise in the pool. Counseling given to her and her family focused on exploring a link between her physical symptoms and psychosocial stressors.

On the ward, Erica did very well. She asked for acetaminophen once or twice the first two days she was there, but by the third day she was medication-free and was eating. However, the psychiatrists treating her did not believe that she or her family accepted a possible link between the alleviation of her headaches and psychologic interventions she was receiving. She was discharged to outpatient psychologic therapy. She was placed in a summer school, where she was able to make up a great deal of the schoolwork she had missed. She was placed in her normal grade the following year, back with her friends and on the sports teams.

Two and a half years later, she is flourishing. She is participating in normal activities, eating, and getting only occasional minor headaches.

This previously well child and her family were devastated by "the headache." Even after all the tests and even hospitalizations she went through, who is to say exactly what the cause of it was?

Here are the salient points about Erica's headache, applicable to other children with long headaches:

1. Chronic headaches place a great strain on a family.
2. Headache treatment requires the cooperation of the child suffering the headaches, her family, and her community.
3. The medications to treat the pain of the headache can cause a number of complications.
4. If psychologic factors are ignored, the most powerful medications may not help.
5. Medical tests into the cause of the headache may not be conclusive, and so sometimes focusing on treatment is more important.
6. Even the most functional children (socially adept, good students, athletes, etc.) can be devastated by long headaches.
7. Nobody should give up. Even a seven-month-long headache such as Erica had can be cured.

• • •

Headache is a challenging problem faced by many children and their families. All headaches (intractable headaches in particular) require patience from the doctor, the patient's family, and the patient himself. So many issues may be involved (both medical and psychological), and symptoms may be difficult to identify and interpret. Diagnosis can be difficult and treatments confusing. However, most sufferers will have a good outcome; most headaches can be successfully treated even if symptoms are severe. Don't let the headaches control your child or your family! Use this book to help you and your child's doctor stay in control of the headaches.

APPENDIX A:
Sample Headache Diary

If desired, this page can be copied and filled out when your child has a headache. The information gathered may help your doctor better diagnose and treat your child.

Date of headache: ______________________________

Day of week: ______________________________

Time headache started: ______________________________

Time headache stopped: ______________________________

Activities during the headache: ______________________________

____

Medication used:

1. ______________________________
2. ______________________________

Time the medication was given:

1. ______________________________
2. ______________________________

Foods and drinks that day: ______________________________

____

____

____

____

Activities that day: ______________________________

____

____

____

____

Stresses or worries: ______________________________

____

____

____

____

____

APPENDIX B: FURTHER RESOURCES

Parents may wish to read the following books for further information:

An Alternative Medicine Definitive Guide to Headaches, Robert Milne, M.D., and Blake More with Burton Goldberg. Future Medicine Publishing, Inc.: Tiburon, Cal. 1997.

Migraine: The Complete Guide. The American Council for Headache Education with Lynne M. Constantine and Suzanne Scott. Dell Publishing: New York, 1994.

Headache in Clinical Practice. Stephen D. Silberstein, Richard B. Lipton, Peter J. Goadsby. Isis Medical Media, Inc., 1998.

Pain in Infants, Children, and Adolescents. Neil Schechter, Charles Berde, and Myron Yaster, eds. Williams and Wilkins, 1993.

Other information can be found through the following groups:

American Council for Headache Education (ACHE)
19 Mantua Rd.
Mount Royal, NJ 08096-3172
Phone: (856) 423-0258 Fax: (856) 423-0082
E-mail: achehg@talley.com Web site: www.achenet.org

National Headache Foundation (NHF)
428 W. St. James Place, 2nd Floor
Chicago, IL 60614-2750
Phone: (888) NHF-5552, (312) 388-6399 Fax: (773) 525-7357
Web site: www.headaches.org

INDEX

About the Author

Sarah Cheyette, M.D., is Board Certified in pediatric neurology and practices in Edmonds, Washington. Pediatric neurologists are specialists in the diagnosis and treatment of headache in children. She completed her residency training in pediatric neurology at the University of Washington and Seattle Children's Hospital and Regional Medical Center, after graduating from medical school at UCLA and undergraduate training at Princeton University. She is a Clinical Instructor at the University of Washington.

Sarah was drawn to pediatric neurology because of the chance to work both with her young patients and their families. She enjoys talking to her patients and their families about how headaches are affecting their lives, and this book is a natural outgrowth of those discussions. In addition, neurologic disorders such as headaches and seizures are in general not well understood, and Sarah enjoys the chance to try to explain what is known about them in a way her patients can easily understand. Over time, she has come to appreciate that pediatric neurology involves not only medical aspects, but psychological and social factors as well. Her greatest satisfaction comes when she can address all of these issues, because it is in this way she feels that she helps her patients the most.

Dr. Cheyette lives in Seattle with her husband, Benjamin, a psychiatrist and research scientist. They have two children, Madeleine Sunshine and Natalie Rose. Two dogs, Seymour and Sydney, are also part of their family.